Creating Your Career Portfolio

At-a-Glance Guide
for Dietitians

Anna Graf Williams Ph.D.

Karen J. Hall

Kyle Shadix, CCC, MS, RD

D. Milton Stokes, RD

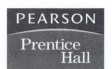

PEARSON
Prentice
Hall

Prentice Hall
Upper Saddle River, NJ 07458

CIP catalog for this record can be obtained from the Library of Congress.

Acquisitions Editor: Vernon R. Anthony
Editorial Assistant: Beth Dyke
Managing Editor: Mary Carnis
Senior Marketing Manager: Ryan DeGrote
Senior Marketing Coordinator: Elizabeth Farrell
Marketing Assistant: Les Roberts
Production Editor: Janice Stangel
Manufacturing Manager: Ilene Sanford
Manufacturing Buyer: Cathleen Petersen
Creative Director: Cheryl Asherman
Senior Design Coordinator: Miguel Ortiz
Development Editor: David E. Morrow
Interior Design & Formatting: Karen J. Hall
Cover Design: Marianne Frasco
Cover Illustration: Eyewire Images

Using a Career Portfolio to Complement Your Professional Development Portfolio

The Commission on Dietetic Registration (CDR) requires a Professional Development Portfolio (PDP) to be developed and maintained by all registered dietitians and dietetic technicians, registered (DTRs), to maintain their registration. It is designed to list participation in continuing professional education activities, such as coursework, presentations, certifications, workshops, lectures and seminars, research, study groups, and self-study.

The career portfolio helps you track and maintain your personal records and documentation that are highlighted in the PDP. The career portfolio stores and presents the documentation you are required to retain by the CDR. Above and beyond that, the career portfolio is a tool for career advancement.

When you assemble a career portfolio, you first take an introspective look at yourself, focusing on your current skills and talents. You then begin to accumulate different types of work samples that prove your skills. Building a career portfolio helps you gain confidence in yourself, while proving to potential employers all that you have to offer. With a career portfolio in hand, you can go into job interviews, reviews, and promotion meetings with proof of your skills and abilities.

Putting together a career portfolio can also assist you in gaining entrance into competitive dietetic internships. After completing a career portfolio, you can fill out the dietetic internship application form with ease. You will have performed a complete self-analysis, having worked through your goals, analyzed your current skills and education, and determined your key responsibilities for jobs and volunteer efforts.

The PDP and the Career Portfolio are complementary tools to your career development.

Anna Graf Williams, Ph.D.

Karen J. Hall

Kyle Shadix, CCC, MS, RD

D. Milton Stokes, RD

Dedication

To all our friends and family who believe in education and know it is not heavy to carry nor a burden to possess. May all your careers be filled with the hope and confidence you find from doing your career portfolio.

Acknowledgments

We would like to thank all the following individuals for helping us complete this project. Without their assistance, we would have never been able to present the materials in such a comprehensive manner. Thank you all for your efforts!

David Morrow

Tracey Morrow

Jennifer R. Eliasi, MS, RD, CDN

Melissa Fabrina, MS, RD, LDN

Rebecca Wright, MS, RD, LD

Renee Zonka, RD, CEC, MBA, CHE

Pamela Charney, MS, RD, CNSD

Martin Yadrick, MS, MBA, RD, FADA

Sari Budgazad, RD, CDN

Stacey B. Freis, MS, RD, CNSD, CDN

CONTENTS

Chapter 7—The Portfolio in Action 129

Chapter 8—A Matter of Style 143

PREFACE

Dietetics is a burgeoning profession. In the last few years, we have witnessed tremendous advancements in food and in nutrition science. Consumers have much to choose from, whether they want to purchase healthier food or locate a practitioner to help with dietary counseling. And more change is right around the corner.

Dietetics professionals work in a variety of areas, including food service operations, hospital inpatient and outpatient clinical nutrition services, private practice, public health, research, academia, and many other fields. The list goes on and continues to grow based on the energy, creativity, and professionalism of those in the field and of those studying to enter the field.

According to the U.S. Bureau of Labor Statistics, employment in the dietetic field is expected to grow about as fast as the average for all occupations through 2012 as a result of an increased emphasis on disease prevention, an increasing public interest in nutrition, and increased emphasis on health education. Baby boomers will boost the demand for meals and nutritional counseling in hospitals, long-term care facilities, prisons, community health programs, and home health-care agencies.

But to get ahead you've got to do something to set yourself apart. Perhaps you have the credentials and the experience, but do you have a way to present yourself to a potential employer? These days it's all about marketing, and with dietetics, we must position ourselves as the most valued source of food and nutrition services. We know we have the skills and training to get the job done, but does a potential employer or a future client know this?

There's one tool that will set you ahead of the competition: the career portfolio. This is a unique process to help you catalog your work experience, accomplishments and awards in an easy-to-use format. With step-by-step instructions presented in a user-friendly format, we demonstrate how you can create your own portfolio. Whether you're a seasoned professional, a new dietitian, or a student working your way toward graduation, this guidebook is for you.

If you're looking to find the right job, stand out among the competition, prove yourself, and feel confident in the interview process, you are ready to create your career portfolio.

Succeed in a tough job market—Use your career portfolio to compete for the job, show your future employer what you are worth, and how you can save them training dollars. Show that employer you are worth the investment!

Stand out—With the help of this book you are going to create a Career Portfolio, a track record of your education and work experiences that you can take with you to a job interview. The portfolio is a zippered three-ring binder containing information about your professional beliefs, experiences, and education. It will contain samples of your work, either in a classroom setting or on the job. The portfolio may also include a list of your skills and abilities. With a portfolio in hand, you can walk into an interview and be able to show the interviewer samples of your work, pictures of projects or community involvement, certificates you've earned, and memberships you have held. Your portfolio will be customized to you, so it will set you apart from everyone else.

Interview with confidence—A portfolio also lets you walk into an interview with more confidence, because while putting it together you'll be examining your goals, writing down your beliefs about work and your career, documenting your strengths, and identifying your weaknesses. By the time you have put together your first career portfolio you should be able to handle those hard interview questions like "Tell me about yourself," "What are your goals for the future?," or "What do you bring to the table for us?"

Start out ahead—Portfolios can do more than boost your confidence in an interview. They can also help you get ahead in the marketplace. A well-crafted portfolio shows employers you have the skills and abilities for which they are looking. We have seen people with portfolios obtain higher starting salaries because they could prove their skills to an employer.

Track your career—Once you have the job, your portfolio doesn't go into a closet until you're looking for another job. Your portfolio changes as you begin to collect and document your work on the job. Then your portfolio serves as proof of your abilities on the job and can be used to track job performance and help position you for advancement.

Creating Your Career Portfolio—At-a-Glance Guide for Dietitians gives you guidelines for creating your career portfolio. In this book you'll find:

- A list of supplies you need to begin this project
- General guidelines for organizing your portfolio
- Detailed discussions of information to be included in different sections
- Pointers on using the portfolio in an interview or job review
- A style guide—containing tips for creating better looking text, photographs, and videos, as well as other ideas for making the production side of the portfolio process run smoothly.

Organization

This book is divided into six sections:

Overview

Chapter 1: "The Portfolio Process"— An overview of the whole process of portfolio development.

Planning and Collecting Materials

Chapter 2: "Planning Your Portfolio"— Tools to help you develop your work philosophy and career goals.
Chapter 3: "The Résumé: An Overview of Your Portfolio"— A look at different types of résumés, both paper and electronic.
Chapter 4: "Proving Your Skills"—How to collect, select, and assemble your work samples, certifications, and community service items.

Putting the Portfolio Together

Chapter 5: "The Assembly"— Putting it all together; producing the portfolio.
Chapter 6: "The Electronic Portfolio"— Creating a digital version of your portfolio for the Internet or distribution on compact disk (CD).

How to Use the Completed Portfolio

Chapter 7: "The Portfolio in Action: Getting the Job"— "Now that I have it, what do I do with it?" Using the portfolio in an interview or to get an internship or co-op experience.

Making the Portfolio Look Good

Chapter 8: "A Matter of Style"— Production tips focusing on making your documents, pictures, and videos look their best.

Quick Reference Materials

Chapter 9: "Resource Guide"— Additional resources to make your career portfolio a success, including:

- Supply list with product numbers
- Emergency assembly instructions
- A list of action verbs for use in résumés
- Skill competencies
- Transferable skill list
- Common job titles and skills for dietitians
- Dietetic work samples
- Common dietetic professional abbreviations
- Sample dietetic internship application
- A list of templates included on the diskette.

We've tried to make this *At-a-Glance Guide* live up to its name. If you like to read books straight through from the beginning, you'll find this book organized in a logical way. If you don't like to read a guide until you need help with a particular step, you're in luck. You don't have to read this book from cover to cover to find helpful information. You'll find an overview to the process in this chapter. Along the way you'll see "Hot Tips", samples, "Ask the Expert" questions, and stories to help you make the most of the career portfolio process.

When you are ready to work on a particular portion of the portfolio, look up the specific section in chapters 2–4 for more information.

For assistance on developing good-looking work samples and documents, refer to Chapter 8, "A Matter of Style."

When you're ready to put your portfolio together, turn to Chapter 5, "The Assembly," or Chapter 6, "The Electronic Portfolio."

Before you go to your interview or job review, reread Chapter 7, "The Portfolio in Action...Getting the Job."

Regardless of how you use this book, you'll find it filled with examples, tips, and ideas that will make the portfolio process truly rewarding.

About the Authors

Anna Graf Williams, Ph.D.

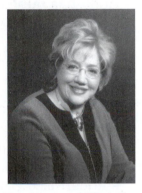

Anna Graf Williams, Ph.D, is a successful business woman and cofounder/senior partner of Learnovation, LLC, an Indianapolis-based publishing and career advancement company. Anna has her roots in food service, strategic planning, and marketing, with her undergraduate degree in consumer and family studies from the University of Illinois and her master's degree in Restaurant Hotel Management from Purdue University. Technology and instructional design work together with curriculum design in Anna's second master's degree to frame her Ph.D in Educational Administration.

Anna has coauthored over 29 books, among whose titles are:

- *Creating Your Career Portfolio At-a-Glance Guide for Students. 3d ed.*
- *Immigrant's Guide to the American Workplace*
- *Family Guide to the American Workplace*
- *Quick Reference Guide to Food Safety and Sanitation*
- *Food Safety Fundamentals.*

Plus 11 videos and a book on tape to name a few!

Anna was formerly one of the youngest full professors in the country having worked at Johnson & Wales University in Providence, Rhode Island. She developed several courses including both graduate and undergraduate diversity management courses. Anna expanded her outcomes assessment expertise through team efforts of standardizing of internship programs.

Anna edited the national career advice publication, *Hosteur,* for hospitality students for five years from 1990-1995. She was also active in Council for Hotel Restaurant Intuitional Education (CHRIE), where she chaired the professional development committee for seven years. Anna is an active member of the Food Service Consultant Society (FSCS), Association for Supervision and Curriculum Development (ASCD), and Small Publishers Association of North America (SPAN).

Anna has published over 250 articles on the topics of career advancement, experiential education, outcomes assessment, hospitality/tourism, and career portfolios. Anna is a popular guest on the nationally syndicated *The Career Clinic*® radio show. Anna is a national public speaker on life skills, career portfolios, and career advancement, having given over 500 presentations. For more details visit the web site www.learnovation.com.

Anna and Karen Hall have focused on career portfolios since 1995, standardizing the process, data collection systems, and standardized curriculum to teach the process. They have written articles and sold tens of thousands of books on the topic. Anna and Karen also co-own Careers with Promise, a company targeting life skills and the delivery of services.

Karen J. Hall

Karen Hall is the "how-to" specialist of the Learnovation, LLC team. As co-founder and senior partner, Karen's focus is in instructional design and product development. Over the past seven years, Karen has spent time refining the mechanics of the career portfolio including the three-hour emergency instructions, templates, and e-portfolio concepts.

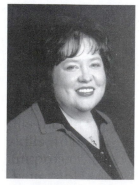

Karen has a master's degree in Instructional Computing from Purdue University where she specialized in instructional design and computer-assisted instruction. Karen has a bachelor's degree in office administration, with emphasis on management information systems from Illinois State University.

Karen has a background in corporate training, from the design and development of materials and documentation to classroom and onsite delivery. She worked as a corporate trainer for a software development company for seven years where she designed and created training programs, materials, and documentation for several different products for the nonprofit industry.

Karen is the coauthor of *Creating your Career Portfolio At-a-Glance Guide for Students. 3d ed.; Creating Your Career Portfolio Practical Exercises; The Family Guide to the American Workplace;* and *the Immigrants Guide to the American Workplace.* She has given many presentations on the Career Portfolio concept and has presented at national conferences and workshops.

When not writing, she is managing the graphic arts and leadership projects in e-training and life skills development for Learnovation, LLC. She is also a co-owner of Careers with Promise, a life skills and services delivery company.

Kyle Shadix, CCC, MS, RD

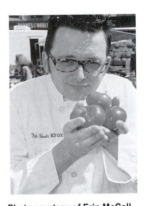

Chef Kyle is a Certified Chef de Cuisine (American Culinary Federation), and received a B.S. degree in Consumer Foods and Nutrition with a minor in Food Science from the University of Georgia, Athens. He spent his junior year abroad in Orleans, France, where he was immersed in French language and culture. Chef Kyle trained at the famed Culinary Institute of America in Hyde Park, New York, where he graduated with honors.

Photo courtesy of Erin McCall

While at New York University, Chef Kyle was a teaching fellow in the Department of Nutrition and Food Studies where he graduated with an M.S. degree in Clinical Nutrition. He completed his dietetic internship at the prestigious Mount Sinai Medical Center (NYC) and God's Love We Deliver. He is a registered dietitian.

Chef Kyle has worked for various companies and institutions including Sloan Kettering Cancer Center, The Food Group New

York City, Daily Soup Company, Gotham Bar & Grill, Mitchel/Abdale Associates for the United Way, Bouley Bakery, personal chef to playwright Terrence McNally and his late partner Gary Bonasorte, and other freelance work.

As an active member in the American Dietetic Association (ADA), Chef Kyle serves on the Membership Advisory Board. Kyle is also the founder and president of the National Organization of Men in Nutrition (NOMIN), a networking group of the ADA. He is a contributing author to the *MinuteMeals* cookbook series (published by Wiley), and he and Milton Stokes, RD, are co-writing *Becoming a Nutritionist*, to be published by Prentice Hall in 2005. Chef Kyle also writes a monthly column for *Today's Dietitian*, a monthly news magazine for nutrition professionals, where he also serves on the editorial advisory board.

Kyle is also the managing partner, along with Milton Stokes, in Culinary Nutrition Consultants, Inc. Please visit www.culinary-nutritionist.com for more on this exciting venture.

D. Milton Stokes, RD

Milton Stokes is a registered dietitian in New York City who works as clinical nutrition manager for Sodexho at North General Hospital. In addition, he's managing partner of his business, Culinary Nutrition Consultants, Inc. (www.culinarynutritionist.com), and a freelance writer.

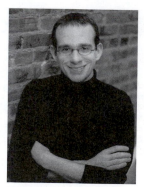

Photo courtesy of Erin McCall

Milton is very involved with the American Dietetic Association and its affiliates, including newsletter writing and editing, book reviewing, and serving in various volunteer and elected positions. His freelance writing has appeared in *Newsweek*, WeightWatchers.com, *Family Doctor*, *American Health and Fitness*, *IDEA Fitness Journal*, *Journal of the American Dietetic Association*, *The Guide to World Nutrition and Health*, and numerous contributions to *Today's Dietitian*. Milton also spent 15 months as a weekly nutrition and health columnist for SlimFast.com.

Milton's undergraduate degree is from Murray State University in Kentucky, and he received a dietetic internship appointment to Yale-New Haven Hospital in Connecticut. He is currently working on his master's of public health and finishing his second book, *Becoming a Nutritionist,* for Prentice Hall.

For more hints, stories, seminar information, questions, and additional resources for the career portfolio, please check out our web site at **http://learnovation.com**. If you have any questions or if we can be of assistance, please feel free to contact us via mail or e-mail.

Learnovation® LLC
My Portfolio
PO Box 502150
Indianapolis, IN 46250

317-577-1190 / Fax: 317-598-0816
E-mail: **portfolio@learnovation.com**

We wish you the best of luck and success in creating your portfolio and developing your career!

THE PORTFOLIO PROCESS

Dietetics is a dynamic profession. Few fields offer as many diverse choices for your career. You can work with people in many different settings and age groups, public and private sectors. You can find a job anywhere in the world—for food and nutrition are a necessary part of our daily lives. You are part educator, part researcher, part lobbyist, and promoter of new ideas and new trends. You work in a field where information and standards change on a regular basis. You are affected by shifting demographics, new medical discoveries, and new trends in food. You work in settings where you are respected for your knowledge and certification, but not necessarily understood. Whether you call yourself a registered dietitian, a nutritionist, a dietary manager, dietetic tech, a nutrition consultant, a nutrition educator, or a research nutritionist, you must work to show people who you are and what you can do.

About Portfolios

In the not too distant past, the word "portfolio" brought to mind two things: a financial investment or stock portfolio, and that big bulky folio of work samples artists carried around to show their work. Today, the portfolio has expanded from the territory of the artist into other professions as well. It is a collection of materials designed to show your work or competencies in a specific area.

The Professional Development Portfolio (PDP)

Continuing education and maintenance of professional credentials is critical in the dietetic field. The Commission on Dietetic Registration (CDR) helps maintain the standards of the dietetic profession by providing specific guidelines for registration in the field. The CDR has established a Professional Development Portfolio (PDP) as a required tool for registration maintenance.

Through the PDP process, you first take a look at yourself and determine your path for your continuing education. Then you record your activities in the PDP. The PDP helps you maintain your credentials.

The Career Portfolio

This book focuses on creating a different type of portfolio: a career portfolio. **Creating a career portfolio follows a similar process, but is designed with a different purpose: to help you promote yourself and advance your career.** A career portfolio is an organized binder of documents that prove your skills and abilities to an employer. In a career portfolio you keep physical samples of your work, skill lists, letters of support or thanks, samples of your volunteer work, details on your education, your professional memberships, your certificates, and awards. It also includes your résumé, a brief bio of yourself and your professional goals. The career portfolio is a complete package that shows who you are and what you can do right now. With your personalized career portfolio in hand, you can go into interview settings with confidence and proof of your abilities. And we are not just talking job interviews here . . . . The career portfolio can also assist you in a dietetic internship interview, a job review, or a promotion review. Use a portfolio anywhere you need to promote yourself.

Competition Is Everywhere

Today, in the extremely competitive job market of the new millennium, many highly qualified people are competing for the same jobs, the same internships, the same opportunities. How can a career portfolio help?

In the Job Market

Employers are looking for new ways to distinguish the excellent people from the average. Having a degree is no longer considered proof of your knowledge, skills, and abilities. Employers are beginning to ask to see results; they want to see physical evidence that shows you possess the abilities you claim; such as managing a tray line, calculating nutrition support regimes, or counseling clients. Individuals are also trying to find new ways to distinguish themselves from the rest of the competitors— to find an edge. The career portfolio is designed to do just that: to provide proof of your abilities and produce a tool that is distinctly you.

The portfolio you create through this process will show the best of your work, your accomplishments, and your skills to eager employers. As the artist's portfolio showed the person behind the art, so will your portfolio show the person behind the work samples. The portfolio also includes other support material including lists of documented skills you possess, volunteer experiences, school involvement, leadership activities, awards and achievements you've earned, letters of recommendation you've received, your goals for your future, and your vision and beliefs for the future of your career in dietetics.

In Dietetic Internships

If you are a currently a student getting ready to apply for a dietetic internship, creating your own career portfolio may be one of the smartest things you can do for yourself. As you plan and assemble your portfolio, you are focusing your goals, documenting your skills, volunteerism efforts, education, and work experiences. You will be able to refer directly to your portfolio to fill in the blanks of your internship form. Writing your letter of interest that goes with the form will be easier if you've already analyzed your experiences and know what you have to offer the organization. Building a career portfolio also builds confidence in yourself. Take your portfolio to the internship interview, customized to the needs of the organization, and you have a powerful tool in your hands—something that can set you apart from the competition.

On the Job

Once you find "the" job, it doesn't mean your portfolio should be thrown into the dark recesses of your closet, only to be resurrected when you want to begin looking for another position. The portfolio is designed to transition with you into your job. As you continue to collect work samples and proof of your experiences on the job, you can turn your portfolio into a useful tool during a job evaluation or promotion review. Think of the impact you will have when you enter a review, fully prepared to show proof of your accomplishments over the last period!

In this chapter, we will provide you with all the basic information you need to create a career portfolio as we answer these questions:

Why do I need a portfolio?

What's in a portfolio?

What supplies do I need to get started?

How do I put it together?

How will I use this in the job search process?

How can I use this in a job review?

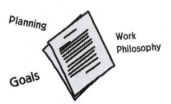

Step 1: Make a career plan.

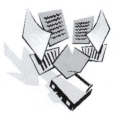

Step 2: Gather work samples, certificates, letters, projects, photos, etc.

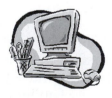

Step 3: Update résumé and references; create support materials.

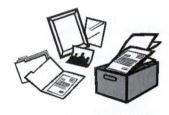

Step 4: Purchase supplies & assemble the portfolio.

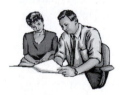

Step 5: Use the portfolio in an interview or review.

The Career Portfolio Process

Why Do I Need a Portfolio?

It's Proof

In an interview or review setting, a career portfolio provides proof of your skills and abilities. Instead of just talking about what you can do during an interview or job review, you can show the person your portfolio—filled with work samples you've created, lists of skills you possess, letters of recommendation, and your professional goals.

An Edge

Recruiters and managers are still not used to seeing portfolios every day. While your portfolio contains samples of your work, it also contains important information about you as a person. You can start interesting conversations that wouldn't be possible without a portfolio in hand. In some cases, having a portfolio can make it easier to stress your strengths in different areas.

It's a Process

The most important thing to remember about portfolio development is that it's a **process**. Of course, the physical portfolio is important, but **the time and effort you put into its development is the true investment in your career**.

Assembling and organizing samples of your work, developing your management philosophy and career goals, and determining the skills and competencies you want to emphasize or obtain in a job situation are key to the production of the portfolio. You can use the portfolio to track the skills you have and the ones you want to possess. As you work through these areas, you begin to examine your experiences and education from different viewpoints. You learn to recognize your strengths and find ways to emphasize these through the portfolio. You are also faced with your weaknesses, and, in the process, you find ways to compensate. This process of examining yourself while developing the portfolio can build your confidence, so there is little, or nothing, an interviewer or recruiter can ask you that you haven't already thought about.

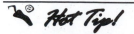

You will find many great work samples for your career portfolio from the activities you complete for your CDR Professional Development Portfolio.

If you are currently working on your Professional Development Portfolio for registration, you will have had the opportunity to look at your career and determine your future goals. You will have many opportunities to acquire work skills and document your abilities as you track your continuing education. Many of these skills and documents can be added to your career portfolio as work samples.

A Disclaimer

Keep in mind we don't claim that having a career portfolio is the ultimate answer to your job search. Jobs aren't going to fall out of the sky at your feet if you just raise your portfolio above your head. Developing a portfolio will help you get organized and prepared for the job market. During this process you will be examining your wants, your skills, your abilities, your strengths, and your weaknesses. This should help you feel more confident in your ability to successfully negotiate an interview. Having a neat, well-organized portfolio also projects a professional image back onto you.

While many of the examples in this book take an interviewing approach to portfolio use, don't forget the portfolio can be a critical tool in job performance reviews and internal job shifting.

What Is a Portfolio?

By this time, you may be telling yourself that it sounds like there's a lot of work involved in this portfolio process. "Analyzing yourself, collecting samples, writing goals . . . can't I just hire someone to do all this work for me?"

The Usual Job Search Tools

First, stop and think about the materials a person usually creates to get ready for the job search process:

- **Résumé**
- **List of references**
- **Cover letter.**

All too often, these are the only materials people prepare and take with them to an interview. We are taught to believe our résumé is the key component of the interview process. Write a good cover letter that explains why you are perfect for this organization, include a nicely formatted résumé that shows education and work experience, include some activities and achievements to trigger their curiosity, and you are done with the process.

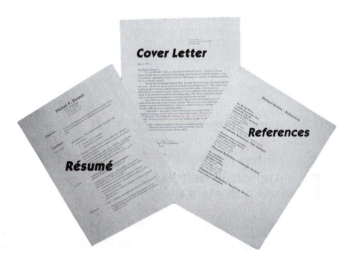

The "usual" interview accessories:
cover letter, résumé, and references.

If you make sure you bring a list of people who will say nice things about you to serve as references, you are ready. Keep in mind the cover letter, résumé, and references are important tools in the job search process. **The résumé and cover letter are the tools you use to get your foot in the door for an interview.** They summarize your abilities and explain why you are well suited to the position. They aren't as helpful during the actual interview, except as a reference for the interviewer.

The Career Portfolio

Now, the person with a Career Portfolio brings a zippered three-ring binder to the interview containing a combination of the following tabbed sections:

Statement of originality	A paragraph stating this is your work and asking them to keep it confidential.
Work philosophy	A brief description of your beliefs about yourself and the food and nutrition profession.
Career goals	Your professional goals for the next two to five years.
Brief biography	A brief narrative of yourself written in third person.
Résumé	A brief summary of your education and experiences.
Skill areas	Tabbed sections containing information on the different types of skills you want to promote such as management, clinical nutrition, patient education, research, communications, etc.
Each skill area may contain:	**Work samples**—Physical examples of your work. Projects, reports, documents, pictures, etc. Highlight case studies, patient education materials, work flow analyses, or other projects completed while in your dietetic internship. Work samples show your skills in this area.
	Letters of recommendation—Letters of support or reference from people who can verify your abilities in this skill area.

Skill sets—Checklists of critical skills related to this area. As you attain different levels of competency with each skill, an instructor or employer can sign off on your ability to perform the skill. These can be pre-existing checklists of skills standardized by an organization or skill sets you create.

Works in progress A brief list of work, activities, projects, or efforts you are in the process of completing.

Certifications, diplomas, degrees, scholarships, and awards Copies of certifications, diplomas, and degrees earned. Copies of special awards and recognitions you have received. Include documentation used to track skills attained for certification. Include a list of any scholarships or awards you have received.

Community service or volunteer experience Work samples, letters of recognition, photos of projects completed, programs and brochures relating to community service projects, and/or volunteer experiences.

Professional memberships/ affiliations and certifications Membership cards, citations, and letters related to professional organizations. Examples might include:

- Dietetic Practice Groups (DPGs)
- American Dietetic Association (ADA)
- American Society for Parenteral and Enteral Nutrition (ASPEN)
- National Restaurant Association's ServSafe Certification
- Certified Diabetes Educator (CDE)
- Board Certified Specialist in Pediatric Nutrition (CSP)

- Certificate of Training in Adult or Adolescent Weight Management Program
- Board Certified Specialist in Renal Nutrition (CSR).

Academic plan of study	A copy of your plan of study that lists courses you have taken to fulfill your degree. Emphasize non-required courses which could enhance your skills such as advanced psychology, exercise physiology, computer applications, etc....
Dietetic internship plan	A copy of your dietetic internship plan or an overview of your internship.
Publications	Any articles you have written, whether for a peer-reviewed journal or your school or company newsletter.
Faculty and employer biographies	Brief descriptions of the people whose names appear throughout the portfolio— who they are and what they do.
References	A list of people who can verify your character, academic record, or employment history.

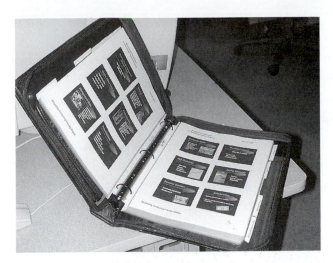

The career portfolio

Now, which person do you think looks more prepared for the interview—the one with the usual tools or a career portfolio?

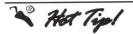 *Hot Tip!*

Many people are too humble to explain their accomplishments. A career portfolio can help them talk about their skills and abilities in an interview setting.

What Supplies Do I Need to Get Started?

The materials you use to create the portfolio serve three purposes:

1. To help organize your documents so you can easily customize your portfolio for a given interview or review period.

2. To make your portfolio look professional. A quick shopping list of supplies, including brands and product numbers, is found in chapter 9, "Resource Guide."

3. To make an easy transition from being a student to becoming a dietetics professional.

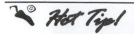

Don't forget to buy extra-wide tabs for the portfolio. Sheet protectors are wider than 3-hole punched paper.

Purchase These Supplies

Here is a list of supplies that will help you to start collecting and assembling your portfolio:

- **Plastic file tote box or flexible file—** Used to store work samples, materials, etc.
- **File folders—**20 to 30 folders.
- **Zippered three-ring notebook—** Cloth, leather, or vinyl with 1-1/2" to 2" rings. Cloth is the cheapest, ranging from $7–$20. Vinyl costs $20–$30, and leather binders often run $60 or higher. All are available at local office supply stores.
- **Sheet protectors—** Clear, plastic, three-hole punched pockets that hold documents and work samples. They protect your portfolio and give it a professional look. Avoid the non-glare variety because they are harder to read.
- **Connected sheet protectors—** Three to five sets of sheet protectors, bound together in sets of five or 10 sheets. These are great for keeping projects and work samples neatly together in your file box. This makes it easier to swap work samples in and out of the portfolio.
- **Tabs—** You can buy printable tabs that adhere to the sheet protectors, or extra-wide three-ring index tabs with labels. Page protectors are wider than ordinary three-ring tabs. You need to find extra-wide tabs made for use with page protectors.
- **Paper—** Use high quality paper when printing your materials. See chapter 8, "A Matter of Style", for suggestions on paper choices.
- **Business card sheets—** Blank sheets of cards are used to create overview cards for work samples.
- **Photo sheet holders—** Plastic sheets that can hold vertical or horizontal pictures.

- **Nameplate or vinyl card holder—** Used on the cover of the portfolio to identify it as your property.
- **Zippered pouch (optional)—** Holds videos.
- **Diskette/CD holders (optional)—** Holds project disks.

A more detailed list, including brands and product numbers, can be found in chapter 9, "Resource Guide."

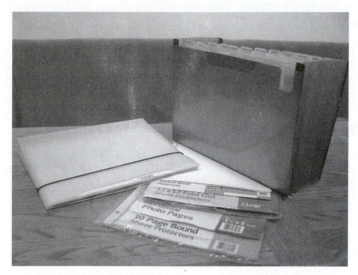

Portfolio supplies

Have Access to This Equipment

A professional portfolio for food and nutrition professionals looks good and feels good. To make this portfolio something you can be proud of, you should plan on using the following equipment when you create documents and work samples to enhance the quality of your career portfolio:

- **Computer—** You should have access to current versions of word processor, graphic presentation, and spreadsheet packages
- **Printer—** Laser or high-quality color ink jet
- **Color flatbed scanner—** Used to scan certificates, work samples, etc.
- **Color copier or color printer—** Used to reproduce work samples, certificates, awards, etc.

- **Film camera or digital camera**— Used for photographing work samples and documenting other activities
- **Video camera**—Videotape yourself in action when necessary.

Things You Don't Need
- **Ink pens**— Do everything on a computer.
- **Three-hole paper punch**— Use page protectors instead of punching holes. Your work will look more professional.
- **Paper clips, staples, and tape**— If you want to connect several pages or display a work sample, use a set of connected sheet protectors.

Planning for Your Portfolio

Getting the supplies together to produce your portfolio is the easy part. Deciding what to put into your portfolio requires planning and organization. Begin by analyzing your strengths and weaknesses. What are you best at? Which skills and abilities do you want to emphasize? Are there things you'd rather not have people ask about, or skills you know you are lacking but would like to have? Taking the time to examine your experiences and abilities will help you focus on your key skill areas you will use in your portfolio. You will also use the planning time to write your work philosophy and career goals. A **work philosophy** gives an employer a unique perspective on you as a person through your personal beliefs about work and your industry. **Career goals** show the employer you have a plan for your life. Chapter 2, "Planning Your Portfolio," focuses on planning your portfolio.

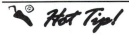

Collect Now— Sort Later! You can decide which samples to use later when you're ready to assemble your portfolio.

Developing Your Résumé

Your **résumé** is a starting point for creating your portfolio. It shows your current skills and experiences and can help you decide what areas to expand on in your portfolio. The résumé acts as a summary of your portfolio. A **brief biography** is a summary of your résumé written in several short paragraphs. It covers your education, what you are currently doing, former jobs that gave you good experience, your memberships, community service activities, and a brief statement about your professional interests. Think about what someone would say if they were introducing you as a group speaker. The brief bio usually comes directly before your résumé in your portfolio.

Collect and Organize Work Samples

You should begin collecting work samples and documents now. You can use projects, reports, photos, letters of recommendation, certificates, newspaper articles, and any materials you have created on the job, in school, in your dietetic internship, or through community service. Start organizing your samples by the type of skills they represent. This will make it easier when it comes time to assemble the portfolio. Chapter 4, "Proving Your Skills," goes into great details about the types of samples to include in your portfolio.

Putting the Portfolio Together

When you are ready to assemble your portfolio, you will gather your supplies, along with a good friend, and select the samples to use.

- Decide what key skill areas you want to focus on and create a **tabbed section** for each. Then pick three or four of your best samples for each area and put them into sheet protectors or photo holders.
- Create an **overview card** for each sample to help a viewer quickly identify the type of sample and what it represents. The card slides into the sheet protector and floats over the top of the sample.

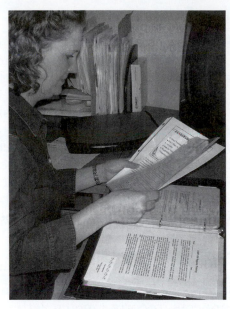

Assembling the portfolio

- Create a **statement of originality and confidentiality** to indicate that this is your work.
- Print out your **work philosophy** and **career goals**, your **brief biography**, your **résumé,** and **references**.
- Create a list of **works in progress** to indicate projects you are working on now for which you have no work samples.
- Create a list of your professional **memberships/affiliations** and create a **Faculty and Employer Bio Sheet** listing information about the people mentioned in your portfolio.
- Put copies of your **certificates, awards,** and **publications** in sheet protectors, along with an **academic plan of study** and **internship plan** if you want to stress your course work.
- Set up and print out the **tabs** and insert them in the dividers.

Chapter 5, "The Assembly," provides more details for putting your portfolio together for presentation. As you are assembling your portfolio, be sure to check Chapter 8, "A Matter of Style," for tips on making your portfolio look its best. Once you put your portfolio together, you're ready to put it to good use.

Using Your Portfolio

So, how do you put the portfolio to work? You can use the portfolio in a job interview, a job review, or to help you create your dietetic internship application.

Using a Portfolio in a Job Interview

Remember, it's your résumé that helps get you the interview. Once you have an interview scheduled, you'll want to make sure the samples in your portfolio show you to the best advantage. Each employer is looking for different things, and you may need to use different work samples to prove different skills. Customize your portfolio for the interview.

Making the Extra Effort

Marcus was excited about his career portfolio and couldn't wait to use it during his first interview with Kalypso Health Services. It was his first opportunity to use his portfolio in an interview, and he just knew he was the right person for the RD position for which he was interviewing. Unfortunately, the interviewer showed very little interest in his portfolio and just seemed to want to talk during his 15-minute interview.

Marcus knew he didn't have the opportunity to share everything he had to offer with the interviewer. He decided to make a spiral bound color copy of his portfolio and send it to the interviewer along with a thank-you letter. It worked! Marcus got a call back and had a much longer second interview where he had the opportunity to answer questions about his portfolio. In fact, Marcus not only got the job, but he got a larger starting salary based on the contents and his explanation of his portfolio.

During the interview you can use your portfolio to answer questions or show examples of your work. Just by having a portfolio along, you can show the interviewer you have organization skills and are focused on your career. Your portfolio can make a lasting impression. Some people have also sent copies of their portfolio along with the thank-you letter after an interview to reinforce their skills, especially when they didn't have a chance to fully use their portfolio during the interview itself.

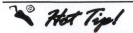

Customize your portfolio to the needs of each interview. Change your work samples and tabbed areas if needed.

Using a Portfolio in a Job Review

The career portfolio is not just a tool for getting a job. If you already have a job and you want to shine in a performance review or want to have an edge in the promotion process, you can use your portfolio to keep track of what you have accomplished and present it in an organized manner.

You can use your portfolio at work to keep track of what you have done and your goals on the job. You can save examples of your work, track your participation in committees and meetings, and use your portfolio to prove your job successes in a job review. Here are some ideas of things to track at work:

- Set goals for each review period and track your achievements. Show how your goals help meet the goals of the company.

- Keep a listing of projects and documents you have completed during the last review period.

- Keep track of the committees and projects you've worked with such as Patient Education Committee, Performance Improvement Committee, Patient Satisfaction Committee, etc.

- Keep copies of thank-you letters and memos that document teamwork or cooperation.

- Include any community service activities in which you have been involved.

- If necessary, update your work philosophy and your career goals, both outside and within the company.
- Ask your supervisor for a six-month review.
- Let your supervisor know well in advance of your review that you are using a career portfolio.
- If your supervisor is new, your portfolio should include highlights of your career since you were hired by the company.

Before Your Review

Let your employer know you have a career portfolio. Talk with your boss and explain the contents of your portfolio. Many promotion and raise decisions are made well before the actual review. Drop off the portfolio a few days before your review so he or she has time to review it. Then discuss it at your annual review.

Megan's Performance Appraisal

Megan has been a registered dietitian for three years and was hoping to get promoted. She let her boss know she wanted to bring her career portfolio to her recent job appraisal and offered her a copy to preview.

During her job appraisal, Megan found her boss to be defensive and somewhat intimidated. Megan was sure it had to do with her portfolio and she asked if she could describe it and explain how she used it. Megan explained to her boss that her portfolio is a "career" portfolio, and she used it to track her performance and abilities on the job. It helped her keep her memberships up to date, organize her skills, and track her goals and objectives.

Megan's boss was so impressed she promoted Megan. She also asked Megan to head up a task force to institute career portfolios for all employees.

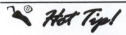

Portfolios can be intimidating to employers if they aren't prepared for them. Explain what your portfolio is and how you are using it before your review.

Using a Portfolio in an Internal Job Shift

The portfolio can be a great help if you are looking to advance or to shift laterally within a company. People job shift inside a company in order to change their responsibilities, find new growth opportunities, or obtain salary increases. An up-to-date portfolio can help you position yourself where you want to be.

Your portfolio needs to contain samples of your accomplishments in your department. You should also include samples that show your management skills of people or projects. Make sure you note any committees or special projects you have been involved in, and highlight your product knowledge and transferable skills.

Using Transferable Skills

Mandy is a registered dietitian at a local hospital. She has always been interested in nutrition and wanted to stay in the job field; however she wanted a job that would allow her to travel and have a more flexible schedule. When a health-care supply sales position opened up at a large therapeutic nutrition company, she decided to overhaul her portfolio and give it a sales twist.

Using the Portfolio to Track Certifications and Complete Your Internship Application

A portfolio is a great tool for managing information. Many people use a portfolio for tracking things they've accomplished on the job; others use it as a way to track progress toward specific certification in the field. Depending on your career path, you may have a structured set of materials that you can put into the portfolio where you can list or mark down what you have accomplished to date. If no formal plan fits, you can create your own forms and lists to track your progress.

Remember, the portfolio isn't just for getting a new job; it's a tool for tracking your skills and abilities. As you obtain new skills, you should add them to the portfolio. Keep this document up to date, and you'll be ready for anything.

You can also use your completed portfolio to help you complete the application for a dietetic internship. Many of the questions you must answer for the internship application will already be in your portfolio. Be sure to take your portfolio with you to any internship interviews.

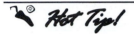 *Hot Tip!*

Use your portfolio in your dietetic internship interviews. Just having it in front of you during a phone interview can be a great confidence builder.

Common Stumbling Blocks to Developing a Career Portfolio

There's no doubt that putting together a career portfolio involves a lot of hard work on your part. Throughout the development of this portfolio process, people kept telling us, "this sounds great but . . . ." Here are some of the common reasons people avoid putting a portfolio together:

- Lack of physical work samples ("I don't have enough stuff to put in a portfolio")
- Unclear personal goals ("What will this do for me?")
- Not sure how to use the portfolio in an interview or review setting
- Lots of jobs to choose from in the career market
- Confusion between a career portfolio and the CDR's Professional Development Portfolio.

The Portfolio in Action

Our friend Jackie has been a registered dietitian for four years and she wanted a new job. Jackie had a solid, formal education and lots of community service background, but she kept blocking when we offered to help her put together the portfolio. This went on for months. Then all of a sudden, one employer said, "Could you do a presentation for us and bring us some of your work to the interview tomorrow?" We followed the guidelines for the "Emergency Portfolio" in chapter 9, "Resource Guide," and helped her create a portfolio for the next day. She admitted that "A portfolio was the best way to organize my work."

Jackie found the process wasn't so bad, and the portfolio worked well in the interview. When we quizzed her about what kept her from doing it earlier, she said, "Most of the résumés I sent out were for jobs where I didn't have an exact match to the company." She felt the portfolio worked best when she could match her work samples to the skills needed by the company.

The story continues. In subsequent interviews she used her portfolio each time. Jackie said, "Most people conducting the interview don't know how to get information out of you. This portfolio stuff works because you can prompt the interviewer to ask better questions." In several interviews, Jackie found the interviewer wasn't very interested in the portfolio at the beginning of the interview, but when she used it to answer a question about her experience, it piqued the interviewer's curiosity enough to look through the whole portfolio. Every time she was asked how well the portfolio worked, she would say, "It blew them away. They were impressed."

We're happy to say Jackie found a job where her talents and experiences could be well used. "I might have still gotten this job without it," she said, "but the portfolio made the interview go more smoothly. The portfolio impressed the interviewers, and it made me a more viable candidate. At my 90-day review I learned I had started about $5,000 higher than average because I had the portfolio and could show them my skills."

I Have Lots of Job Offers so I Don't Need a Portfolio . . .

"The job market is real good right now and I have lots of offers." If this sounds like you—congratulations! You may not need a career portfolio to get the job, but you can still use a portfolio to get a better offer. With a portfolio, you have your professional goals spelled out and you have physical proof of your abilities. You can use these features to get more money or better benefits. The money being offered may be preset, but the benefits package can often be expanded for secondary benefits, such as non-insurance and retirement benefits.

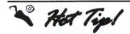 *Hot Tip!*

Use a portfolio as a bargaining tool when you have lots of job offers.

There is something about the portfolio process which causes you to reflect on who you are, what you want to do, and to search out what you are good at doing. Using the portfolio process for upping the offer in the interview sets you up to use it on the job during your performance appraisals or year-end reviews.

Upping the Offer

Pam received three job offers and developed a portfolio to help justify her negotiations for benefits and perks. She used her portfolio to demonstrate her abilities and her need for professional development. Each of these companies agreed to pay for her professional memberships and one three-day professional meeting. This would save her an average of $1,200 out-of-pocket expenses per year. She was also able to convince her eventual employer to purchase an additional copy of the software they used in the office for home use. This made her job easier by having the same software at home to do her work.

I Am Already Doing a CDR Portfolio . . .

The CDR Professional Development Portfolio is designed to help you develop and track your continuing education plan to maintain your dietetic registration. You must log your attendance and participation in continuing education activities in your portfolio.

A career portfolio is designed to help show your current skills and abilities in a way that helps you to promote yourself in a job search or job review setting. It is very much a hands-on tool that you can use to physically show people your work. The focus of your career portfolio is career advancement. Many of the things that are tracked in the CDR portfolio may actually appear in your career portfolio. Copies of your goals, certificates, proof of attendance at workshops, copies of presentations given to a group, or community service photos would all be appropriate work samples to include in your career portfolio. The career portfolio is not focused just on your continuing education needs, but on showing all the skills and knowledge you have right now.

If You Need a Portfolio Now . . .

"Oh, it won't take that long to put it together."

"I have one that I used last time."

"My interview is tomorrow and I have to do all this before I can start on my portfolio?"

"Help, I have an interview tomorrow and they asked me to bring work samples!"

If you've just purchased this book and want to put together a portfolio for an interview tomorrow morning, or if you've had this book for a while and suddenly your interview is upon you, there's still hope. Based on several frantic experiences of our own, rest assured you can put together a basic career portfolio in three hours if you have a computer, printer, and a friend to help. See chapter 9, "Resource Guide," for all the details on creating an emergency portfolio.

Read On

You now have the basic ideas necessary to create your portfolio. In the following chapters, you will learn how to plan and organize your portfolio and make it a personalized tool for career success.

We've organized these sections as you would position them in the completed portfolio. This doesn't mean you will be developing your materials in this order; quite the contrary, you have to make the most of the opportunities at hand. You'll probably be saving projects and papers or securing signatures for skill areas long before you focus on your résumé. Refer to Chapter 5, "The Assembly," for tips on organizing and creating the portfolio.

Keep in mind as you continue through this book that a portfolio provides:

Insight into you as a person

- Statement of Originality & Confidentiality
- Work philosophy
- Goals.

A summary of your portfolio

- Brief biography
- Résumé.

Proof of your abilities

- Skill areas containing:
  - Work samples
  - Letters of recommendation
  - Skill sets
  - Community service/volunteerism
  - Certifications, awards, scholarships, degrees, training, and diplomas
  - Works in progress.

Your commitment to your own personal and professional growth

- Professional memberships/affiliations
- Professional development plans.

Reference materials

- Internship plan
- Academic plan of study
- Faculty and employer bios
- References.

Once you've completed your portfolio you'll feel a great sense of accomplishment. You've created a tool that can help you through the job search and can go forward with you in your career.

 Taking Action!

Start working on your career portfolio now!

- Get a box or file and start saving work samples
- Track down your existing work samples: documentation, certificates, awards, etc.
- Review the list of supplies you need to create a portfolio
- Begin to plan ahead for getting letters of recommendation and finding people who will serve as your references.

CHAPTER 2

PLANNING YOUR PORTFOLIO

One of the exciting things about a career in dietetics is the wide variety of work environments. You can choose from health-care facilities, commercial food services, wellness centers, schools and universities, research companies, sales, marketing, and general practice. If you want to know the possibilities, go into a job search web site, such as www.monster.com and type in registered dietitian. See what types of companies are listed. For just this reason, you need to plan your portfolio for the area or job you are targeting. You can customize your portfolio for the specific occupation you're using it in. This is when you begin to evaluate your work philosophy and establish goals for your career. This chapter will provide you with the mechanics and several tools for generating the pieces you need in your portfolio. You analyze current and yet-to-be acquired skills. This is where you design your career. Keep in mind your career is more than a job—it's the paths those jobs take.

Designing Your Career

The first step to developing your career goals is to take an in-depth look at your skills, interests, and abilities from a professional and personal perspective. Understanding and identifying the different skills you have can help you be better prepared for a job or keep you on track for a promotion. Knowing what you have to offer an employer is important, and you may have more going for you than you think! Once you know where you're going, you can use some techniques to help you develop your action plan.

Identifying Your Skills

If you're in school, you are constantly learning new skills. At the beginning of every new class, your teachers usually start by reviewing the goals and objectives for the class. You know what you will be learning and what skills you should have by the time you finish the class. Whether you're taking a food science class or medical nutrition therapy, you are gaining skills in that area. In your job, you are learning and expanding your skills as you advance in your career.

Skills are often broken down by the type of skill you are learning. **Hard skills** relate to practical skills, like the ability to plan a menu for people with diabetes or an understanding of pediatric nutrition. Most classes are geared to learning a set of hard skills. The following chart gives a sample of the hard skills dietitians must have to be registered.

A Sampling of Hard Skills

Food Preparation

- Menu formulation
- Food preparation
- Purchasing.

Food safety

- Knowledge of health, safety, and issues related to food consumption trends
- Nutrient composition of foods, food additives, food allergies and hypersensitivities
- Naturally occurring toxins, pathogens, pesticides, biotechnology-derived foods
- Irradiated foods
- Food laws and regulations.

Assessment

- Assessment and screening techniques
- Medical record reviews
- Care plan development
- Documentation techniques.

Nutrition in disease

- Physiological and biochemical aspects of nutrition metabolism
- Biochemical and physiological principles of nutrition for sport, obesity, eating disorders, respiration, alcohol metabolism, inborn errors, immunity, cancer
- The nervous system and trauma.

Soft skills consist of a broader range of skills related to your personality and attitudes. Examples of soft skills include self-confidence, communication skills, teamwork skills, tolerance, discipline, management, etc. Working on a team project, problem solving a process, leading a meeting, and being able to make decisions are some of the soft skills you can gain from a class without knowing it. They are often thought of as hidden skills, but they are some of the most important skills you can have. Employers are always looking for people with a certain set of hard skills, but when they have good soft skills to go with them, they can be a powerful combination in a good employee. Take a look at the following list to see just what kinds of skills employers are seeking. You can use your portfolio to promote many of these soft skills.

Soft Skills Employers Seek

Teamwork

Being a good team member means:

- Putting the good of the team ahead of yourself
- Respecting others' opinions
- Hearing people out
- Involving everyone in finding solutions to problems.

Presentation skills

- Leading a meeting
- Promoting an idea to the boss
- Giving your thoughts in a union meeting.

Communication skills

- Answering the phone
- Writing e-mails
- Putting together a proposal
- Interacting with co-workers and customers
- Being a good listener
- Giving and receiving feedback.

Leadership

- Heading up a project
- Training others
- Delegating
- Negotiating
- Managing conflict
- Planning
- Setting priorities
- Organizing skills.

Other Soft Skills

- Problem solving
- Multi-tasking
- Thinking quickly
- Ability to make decisions
- Customer service
- Courtesy
- Ability to work with people from different cultures
- Work ethic
- Self-discipline.

Ask the Expert
Identifying the skills I need

Q. How do I know what specific skills I need to prove to get the job I want?

A. A good way to identify what skills you may need to prove is by reviewing job postings for the entry-level position and future positions you may seek. Most potential employers will indicate what skills they value in their job advertisement or job description. Usually, after reviewing a variety of job postings, you will see a pattern of skills desired by potential employers.

Transferable Skills

Transferable skills are the skills you've gathered through various jobs, volunteer work, hobbies, sports, or other life experiences that can be used in your next job or new career. Transferable skills are important to those who are facing a lay-off or looking for a different job, new graduates who are looking for their first jobs, and those re-entering the work force after an extended absence. Transferable skills are skills you can use in a variety of industries and settings. A person with management skills can transition from a career in clinical nutrition management to a career as vice president of nutrition and food service operations. An RD with a hobby of marathon running could use his running knowledge to relate to clients in a sports nutrition and wellness center. Another person took her skills as a registered dietitian and moved into a position in diabetic equipment sales. Begin to identify your skills and how they can be used in different ways. What else can you bring to the table in terms of expertise? Are you a subject matter expert in any fields? The ability to speak a second language could be the asset that sets you apart from other candidates and gets you the job.

Transferable Skills

- Verbal communication
- Nonverbal communication
- Plan and organize
- Counsel and serve
- Create and innovate
- Written communication
- Train/consult
- Interpersonal relations
- Leadership
- Management
- Financial
- Administrative
- Analyze
- Construct and operate
- Research.

Transferable skills can be hard or soft skills. If you can drive a semi truck, a hard skill, you can also drive a delivery van. If you can coach a softball team, you have soft skills that can be used when training people on the job. Look at the above list of transferable skills that employers like to see. Notice how many of the skills listed are soft skills. Check out chapter 9, "Resource Guide," for a detailed list of transferable skills.

Strengths, Weaknesses, Opportunities, and Threats to Your Career (SWOT)

Once you've identified your skills, you need to take a look at some of the other factors that affect your career choices. A SWOT analysis is a method of looking at the **S**trengths, **W**eaknesses, **O**pportunities, and **T**hreats in a specific situation. SWOT started as a way to analyze nonprofit organizations and has, in the last 30 years, transitioned to business planning as well as personal planning. You can use a SWOT analysis to help explore issues, skills, strengths, and weaknesses you have in your career search. In this case, we can apply the process to your career.

Strengths and weaknesses are personal to you; they are things you can control. Take a look at the skill of analyzing a patient's diet. One person may list dietary analysis as a strength, yet another person may list the same skill as a weakness.

You control your ability to analyze a patient's diet; therefore it would be listed as either a strength or a weakness. How skilled you are is something you can control because you can choose to focus a specific skill to enhance it, or you can choose to accept the skill as a personal weakness; either way, you control it.

Opportunities and threats are things in your environment that you can't control. Opportunities are positive things that work to your advantage, whereas threats are negative factors that could be a potential setback to your plans. A person considering a career as a registered dietitian might list the prestige and salary as an opportunity, whereas the cost of schooling and the length of time needed to obtain a degree and certifications could be listed as a threat. These items are listed as opportunities or threats because they cannot be directly controlled.

The SWOT analysis is the part of the process where you really size up what you have to offer. When doing a SWOT, you should look at all the characteristics that influence your professional and personal life.

Take a look at this shopping list of characteristics for things you **can control**:

- Skills in your field
- Supervision/management/leadership abilities
- Types of teams
- Communication (written, electronic, verbal, and non-verbal)
- Technology (types of software and projects)
- Social (professional and service groups)
- Personal areas such as community service.

Give some additional consideration in your analysis to those things you **do not control**:

- Economy/demand for jobs
- Social trends (health, transportation, and e-commerce)
- Political (government or workplace)
- Technology (software and hardware changes)
- Advancement availability (career path, age and experience of those around you)
- Location (job, geography)
- Workplace culture (work ethic, family values, and uses of power)
- Required education (certifications, etc.).

The following two pages show a completed SWOT analysis for a dietetic student currently in an internship. This student analyzed her personal strengths and weaknesses as well as the opportunities and threats she could face as a dietitian in the field.

 Template

A blank set of career SWOT sheets are available on the companion diskette **(SWOT Analysis.doc)**. Print out the pages and complete your own SWOT analysis.

SWOT Analysis—Your Career

Things You Control

Rank	Your STRENGTHS	Your WEAKNESSES	Rank
	Skills related to your field	**Skills related to your field**	
3	Patient education with known materials	Patient assessment without criteria	2
1	Dietary analysis	Counseling new patients	3
4	Food safety certified	Biochemistry	1
2	Identifying health ailments		
	Management	**Management**	
1	Planning for the overall operation	Multi-tasking	1
3	Time management	Financial management	3
2	Organization	Record keeping	2
4	Project management		
	Teamwork	**Teamwork**	
2	Team player	Goal focused	1
1	Leadership	Handling conflict	2
3	Sharing tasks		
	Communication	**Communication**	
3	E-mail	Written reports	2
2	Phone	Communication with superiors	1
1	Patient		
4	Delegation		
	Technology - (software, Internet telecommunications, etc.)	**Technology - (software, Internet telecommunications, etc.)**	
4	Microsoft Word	Microsoft Access	1
3	Microsoft Excel	MAC programs	2
1	Nutribase		
2	The Food Processor (ESHA)		
5	Internet research for patient education		
	Social	**Social**	
1	Patience	Asking for help	1
2	Responsive to patient needs	Networking	2
3	Following directions		
	Personal Areas - Family/Friends/ Spiritual/Financial/Health	**Personal Areas - Family/Friends/Spiritual/ Financial/Health**	
2	Loyalty	Follow-through with personal goals	1
4	Value multiculturalism		
1	Dependable		
3	Trustworthy		

SWOT Analysis—Your Career

Things You Don't Control

Rank	OPPORTUNITIES you can use	THREATS that face you	Rank
	Economy/Demand for Jobs	**Economy/Demand for Jobs**	
1	High demand for skilled dietitians	Economic pressure on employers	1
2	Demand expected to grow as fast as the average		
	Social Trends	**Social Trends**	
3	Low-carb diets	Diet trends shift	1
2	Obesity levels on the rise	Sports/health issues for baby boomers	2
1	Overall need for diet care		
4	Poor diets in children		
	Political (government or workplace)	**Political (government or workplace)**	
1	Government programs supply jobs	1 in 5 jobs are provided by state/local government	1
2	Nutrition is a hot political topic		
	Techonology	**Techonology**	
1	Improved technology can make job functions easier	Technological advances require new learning	1
	Advancement Availability	**Advancement Availability**	
1	New areas that need dietitians	Certifications take time to obtain	1
	Location (job, geography)	**Location (job, geography)**	
1	Variety of work environments	Kitchens can be warm/congested	1
2	Positions available country-wide		
3	International availability		
	Workplace Culture	**Workplace Culture**	
1	Holidays off	Weekend work	1
2	40-hour workweek/plus	On feet for most of the day	2
	Required Education	**Required Education**	
2	Registered when education complete	Time consuming	2
1	Internships prepare for real life	Certifications difficult to obtain	1
		Internships are time consuming	3

Look at your skills and abilities in your personal and professional life. Where are you now? What are your strengths? What are your weaknesses? List them under the major headings; then rank them from the strongest to the weakest. Once you know your strengths and weaknesses, you will know what areas to promote and can formulate your goals for where you would like to be.

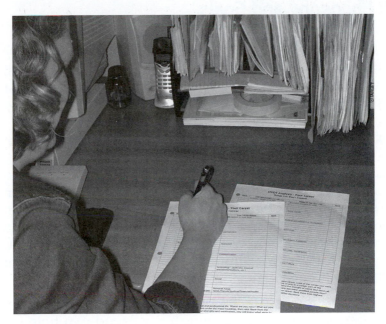

The SWOT analysis can help you focus your career goals.

Ask the Expert

I want to be promoted

Q. I am currently employed as a dietary aide but want to be considered for a promotion to dietetic technician during my next performance review. What can I be doing now to be considered for this position when it becomes available?

A. Begin by gathering evidence of your skills and abilities that would make you successful as a dietetic technician. Perhaps you have had a job in the past where you were responsible for higher-level functions, or you have been asked to perform some duties that are typically handled by dietetic technicians.

What work samples would you have from these experiences? You also need to ensure that you have completed all the educational requirements needed to be eligible to sit for the exam. You may want to consider volunteering for some tasks or activities with any associations you belong to that would help you prepare for your next step.

Work Philosopy and Goals

Now that you have taken a look at your skills and you've at least thought about doing a SWOT analysis, you're ready to create two of the first documents that will appear in your portfolio, your work philosophy and your goals.

Work Philosophy

A work philosophy is a statement of your beliefs about yourself, people, and your outlook on life in your industry. Your work philosophy is often used by an interviewer to see if you match a company's corporate culture. After reading this statement, a potential employer should know whether you would fit the "style" of the organization. Your work philosophy might also be called a management philosophy.

Make sure you have a friend to assist you when you're ready to develop your work philosophy. Your friend can help you take your beliefs and the ideas that you have internalized and verbalize them on paper. Many people know in their hearts what they believe, but they've never put it into words.

Here's the work philosophy of one graduating student:

Work Philosophy

- The customer always comes first.
- Financial and operational controls must be clear to all members of the company.
- Technology will be critical in reaching the client and communicating within the company.
- I want to be part of a winning health-care team.

What you need to know about your philosophy...

- **Think about it—** Don't expect to "whip out" a work philosophy or personal mission statement in 10 or 20 minutes. It usually takes a few days worth of thought and reflection before the "final draft" is ready.

- **Place your most important belief first—** Your work philosophy should be unique to you, communicate who you are, and what makes you different from others who may want the same position.

- **Length—** Your work philosophy should be one to four sentences in length and should address your beliefs and your outlook on people.

- **Use bullets—** Consider using bullet points for added clarity.

- **Have a friend review it for clarity—** After you have it on paper, ask a few friends to read it for clarity—not approval. Remember, your work philosophy is never right or wrong; it represents your key beliefs and values.

 Template

Use the **Work Philosophy and Goals.doc** file on the companion diskette as a starting point for developing your own portfolio.

Goals

If you don't have goals, your career will be one reaction after another. With your career goals in mind, you can determine which opportunities to accept and which to decline. Your goals set a direction for your career and are general in nature. The goals in your portfolio should focus on the professional achievements, skills, and knowledge you want to acquire over the next several years. Companies use these goals to anticipate your developmental needs and interests. They also show management and recruiters that you do indeed have a plan for your future.

Here again, a friend can help you develop your goals. He or she can ask questions that make you think about your goals and can help make sure your goals make sense.

Making Your Goals Work

- **Plan your goals for two to five years from now—** When writing goals, think ahead several years. What do you want to be doing in two years? What do you want to have accomplished four years from today? Goals written for one year or less are often too narrow in focus and usually concentrate on learning a new position rather than planning for the future. You should also make sure your goals are not so specific as to imply only a narrow interest in dietetics or in a specific job. If you are starting in an entry-level position, think about the job you want to be doing in two to three years. Goals can help share your vision for where you will fit in the organization in the future.

- **Make your goals measurable—** Your goals should be specific enough that you will know when you've achieved them. We measure goals in terms of time, money, and resources.

    Too broad:
    "To expand my technical knowledge."

    Good:
    "To develop my nutrition analysis skills by attending a class on Nutribase by May 2006."

- **Goals are different from career objectives—** Career objectives are broad and set a direction for your career. Goals are more specific; they include shorter-range objectives that are measurable.
- **Write three to five goals—** If you only write one or two goals, you may appear unfocused and give the impression you're not really interested in advancing your career.
- **Don't make your goals too personal—** Goals such as losing weight or winning a marathon can alienate your interviewer; it may give the person more information than he/she may want to know about sensitive topics. Keep your goals professional and related to your career.

Here is a sample of goals that are appropriate for individuals just starting their careers:

Two-Year Goals

- To be assistant clinical nutrition manager
- To hold at least one active professional membership
- To volunteer in a food pantry
- To earn the customer service award
- To further develop my computer application skills as they apply to controlling costs
- To apply my creativity to develop new menus.

 Template

Use the **Work Philosophy and Goals.doc** file on the companion diskette as a starting point for developing your own goals and your philosophy.

Building Your Portfolio Plan

Take a look at all the skills you have and the results of your SWOT analysis and build your portfolio plan. It is critical to your success to understand what you have as skills and characteristics and to create a vision for what you want to do in your profession.

Taking time to evaluate your career and focus your goals will help you in the next phase of the portfolio—putting your résumé together and finding and gathering the proof of your abilities. Don't underestimate the importance of the activities in this chapter. Having the focus will help you determine how to build skill sections of your portfolio and help you focus on producing a valuable tool.

 Taking Action!

Planning can be hard work!

- Print the SWOT analysis template from the CD and do a SWOT analysis on your career. See what you learn.

In your current job:

- Find your job description and expand or enhance it to reflect what you really do.
- Look at opportunities and job paths available in your company.

In your school work:

- Look at each class you are taking and determine the skills you will have when you finish the course.

In your career portfolio:

- Write your work philosophy. Use the template included on the CD as a place to start.
- Write your three-year goals using the same template file.

CHAPTER 3

The Résumé: An Overview of Your Portfolio

Everyone knows about résumés. They are the most common vehicle used in the job-hunting process and are used to convey information about your experiences and qualifications. A résumé usually contains a summary of your education, work experiences, and qualifications for a position. When used in conjunction with your portfolio, the résumé serves as a spring-board for introducing your portfolio into the conversation. It also provides a summary of the contents of the portfolio.

This chapter gives general suggestions for creating your résumé. If you want specific details, you'll find a wealth of information on the Internet. At the end of this chapter, we've included some good web sites to help guide you in the process of creating your résumé and making it look its best.

What Goes into Your Résumé?

Creating a résumé is often a daunting task for anyone about to pursue a job search. It is the crucial tool needed to get an interview and creating it can be a painful experience. There is so much conflicting information about résumés available today. Here are some of the most common questions people ask: "Can it be more than one page?" "Does my education or experience go first?" "What do I do about gaps in my experience?" "How do I make myself look really good without bragging?" "How do I make them see my résumé in the huge pile on the secretary's desk?" "How far back should I go with my experience?" "What if I'm switching fields?" "What if I don't have all the qualifications they are looking for?"

Résumé Basics

If you are just entering the work force, your résumé will look very different from that of a person who has had several years of experience in his or her field. In general, most résumés have a combination of the following sections:

Career objective/career summary— A **career objective** is an overview of the kind of work you want to do: a one- or two-sentence summary of your career goals. If you have been in the work force for several years, you may want to use a career summary. The **career summary** consists of two to three sentences which briefly outline your career history.

Education— Include any formal education, degrees obtained and in progress, the institution, dates attended, and the focus of your degree(s).

- The less experience you have, the more you need to build up your education. You might consider listing classes you took which are relevant to the field you are entering.

- List any formal education or training programs you have taken which relate to your field.

- List your most recent achievements first.

Work experience or skills— Include your job title, name of the organization, dates employed, and an overview of your skills and experience.

- If your work experience is stronger and/or more recent than your education, list your work experience first.

- List your accomplishments and/or responsibilities with each position.

- List your most recent experience first.

Professional memberships and services, awards received— Include memberships and awards that demonstrate your abilities, enhance your leadership, or document your skills. Examples of awards might include Recognized Young Dietitian of the Year (RYDY), Outstanding Dietetic Student, Emerging Dietetics Leader, etc.

Community service— List organizations and your involvement with them.

Contact information— Include your name, address, phone number, fax number, and e-mail address.

Let people know you have a portfolio— Your résumé also needs a line at the bottom of the last page indicating that your portfolio is available for review:

Career Portfolio and References available for review

Organizing Your Résumé

There are several standard ways of organizing a résumé depending on your experiences, skills, and target industry:

- **Chronological résumés—** Information is organized by date. Information is listed in order of time elapsed, with the most recent experiences first. This is the most common and straightforward résumé format.

- **Functional résumés—** This type of résumé is designed to highlight accomplishments and specific skills. It is organized by the different kinds of skills you can perform, such as management skills, marketing, finance, etc.

- **Performance résumés—** This résumé type is a combination of the chronological and functional approaches. You list employment information in a chronological format, then organize the skills you've developed in each position in order to highlight your accomplishments.

- **Focused résumés—** This résumé lists only those jobs you've had which directly relate to the specific area you are targeting. This format is often used by large corporations to track performance and skills within their own organization. If you are looking for promotion within a company, this format may suit your needs. This format is not as popular because it is very specific.

- **Government résumés—** If you are interviewing for a government position or with a company that contracts with the government, you may be asked to submit a standardized résumé, laid out in a specific format. They are usually narrative in nature, and should use terms from standardized job descriptions and other government documents.

Here's a résumé of a graduating student:

Melissa Lyons

100 West Way – City, State 12345 – Work: (123) 456-7890, Home: (987) 654-3210
email:mlyons@provider.com

OBJECTIVE

Student seeking a position that is challenging and educational in a nutrition related field.

EDUCATION

Bachelor of Science, Nutrition Science 6/00
University of California, Davis

WORK EXPERIENCE

01/03-Present   **Student Volunteer**, CRP W.I.C. Sacramento. Assisted with various one-on-one counseling sessions with dietitians and nutrition assistants by observing and translating. Attended various nutrition education classes for WIC participants. Became familiar with ISIS database used for tracking WIC participants. Developed an Access database and assisted with researching participants for a breastfeeding study. Assisted with developing a class outline and reading materials for raising participant awareness about local Farmer's Markets.

09/02-Present   **Student Intern**, California State University, Sacramento Health Center. Responsible for assisting students with health and wellness inquiries. Performed diet analysis on student three day food records. Assisted with various presentations, health fairs, promotions regarding nutrition and health related issues. Developed handouts, posters and bulletins for promoting health and wellness. Conducted presentations in student dormitories to promote low-fat living.

10/99-Present   **Student Assistant**, California Department of Education, Commodity Distribution Unit. Duties include: Researching and preparing nutrition fact sheets for U.S. Department of Agriculture (USDA) commodities distributed. Contact agencies by phone to monitor current participation in the Donated Food Program. Keep track of food shipments using access databases. Assist with unit PowerPoint presentations. Review and update state processing agreements, unit documents and manuals. Do continuous filing of incoming documents. Survey recipient agencies regarding program modifications/needs. Compile survey information into reports for USDA. Coordinate food ordering for the Commodity Supplemental Food Program. Provide clerical support to staff on a daily basis.

SPECIAL SKILLS

- Able to read, write, and speak Spanish fluently
- Experienced with Microsoft Word, Excel, Access and PowerPoint
- Familiar with office equipment
- Able to type 55 wpm

CLUBS & ACTIVITIES

- Member of the Food and Nutrition Club/Dietetics at California State University, Sacramento

Career Portfolio and References available for review

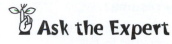

Ask the Expert

Résumé Do's and Don'ts

Q. How do I choose which organizational style to use?

A. It depends on your audience and your experience. People with limited experience and education should use the chronological layout. If you have more experience and/or education and want to emphasize your skills or course work, use a performance résumé. That way you can list your courses and highlight skills obtained from your jobs. If you have been in the work force for several years and are looking to highlight your skills for a promotion or applying for a job where you are emphasizing your experience, use the functional résumé.

Q. What if I am short on education or work experience?

A. If you are coming out of college and looking for a starting position, you'll want to emphasize your course work as well as any internship you may have completed. Highlight the classes that related to your major and indicate the types of skills you gained from the courses. Use your internships, community service, or volunteer work you have done that will prove real-world experience. You may also choose to join additional professional organizations that will get you connected to other people in the field.

Q. Do I put education or work experience first?

A. If you have education but limited work experience, list education first. If you have been in the work force for several years, list experience first. You decide which is stronger: your education or your work experience.

Q. Do I list everything I've done?

A. If you have limited work experience, list it all. If you have had a variety of short-term positions, list the jobs that are relevant to the position for which you are applying. Some experts recommend leaving off any experiences older than 10 years, but if the experiences have value and add to your employability in the current position, go ahead and list them.

Q. What do I do if I have time gaps in my résumé?

A. If you're talking about timelines where you were unemployed for a period of time, leave the gap and be prepared to talk about it if the question arises in an interview.

Q. What do I do if I have skill gaps in my résumé?

A. If you have skill gaps, where you don't have all of the qualifications for the position but you are applying anyway, you will want to emphasize your strengths and your ability to learn new skills. The cover letter that goes with the résumé may be the best place to address this. Be sure to use keywords specific to the industry so your résumé will have a better chance of getting to the "interview" pile.

Q. What if I don't have any awards?

A. It's OK if you don't have any awards to display in your portfolio. You can use your work experience and education to promote your skills and abilities. However, awards can be helpful when they are incorporated into your portfolio. Awards can be secured through many avenues: from a job, being on a committee with a professional organization in your field, or from any community service activities you are involved in. Volunteering for leadership roles is one of the best ways to get awards.

Q. Should I list all the professional memberships I hold?

A. Holding professional memberships tells employers you are committed to your career field. It is appropriate to list all the memberships you hold, but more important, highlight the activities you are involved with in those organizations. There is a difference between simply being a member of a professional organization and being an active member. Volunteering for fund-raising efforts, assisting with conference planning and execution, and holding offices with an association are all good ways to show active membership.

Q. Should I list my references on the résumé?

A. Most employers do not contact references until you have been interviewed and you are being considered for the position. Besides, you may need all that room to list skills gained from course work or job experiences. Create a separate reference sheet and indicate on your résumé that your career portfolio and references are available upon request. Include a copy of the references in your portfolio and keep an individual copy available to give to the interviewer if it is requested.

Q. I've heard that my résumé should fit on one page. Can I go over one page in length?

A. As a general rule, if you are just out of school, you should be able to keep your résumé to one page. If you have more experience you can expand it. Even the most experienced person should keep his or her résumé to three pages. Your résumé can be longer than one page, but be sure the information you include is a good representation of you. Some experts say you should always fill the extra pages. Don't have a one-and a half-page résumé. Today, more résumés are being sorted and processed electronically, where a computer program scans for certain keywords. You may benefit from listing key skills and abilities you have gained from your experiences, and that can take up more space.

Q. What is the difference between a résumé and a curriculum vitae? Which one should go in my career portfolio?

A. A résumé is a summary of your education and career history. It is meant to give potential employers a brief summary of your experience and a list of your skills. A curriculum vitae (CV) lists every job, degree, publication, and just about everything you have accomplished in your academic and career life. Most employers, when seeking out potential candidates, will want to see your résumé. If you are seeking higher-level positions, it is appropriate to have your CV available. However, neither of them "document" your skills and abilities the way a portfolio does. Supplying real-world work samples that prove your skills and abilities in a career portfolio is what gives you an edge over other candidates.

Q. Can I use a fancy type style and paper to help my résumé stand out from the rest?

A. With many job openings generating hundreds of applications, employers are looking to technology to help them deal with the volume of applicants. They will often scan a résumé into electronic format and then use a software program to scan for certain keywords in the résumé. One of the problems with fancy type styles is that they don't scan well. The software is used to dealing with plain type styles and can mess up on fancy ones. The last thing you want is to have your résumé scanned and your name come in wrong because you have it in a funky font. The same rule goes for paper. Using paper with shaded or mottled backgrounds can cause the scanner to mis-read words.

Your best option is to use a readable font, on high quality white paper. Lay out your résumé with plenty of white space in an attractive format and use appropriate keywords to set your résumé apart. Check out chapter 8, "Style Guide," for more details on making your résumé look great.

 Template

Most word processing programs such as Microsoft Word and Word Perfect include templates for creating résumés. We suggest you use these templates as a starting point for creating your own résumé.

Choosing the Right Words

Regardless of the style of résumé you choose to create, you should describe the skills and experiences associated with your jobs and education. Using the right words to capture experience can sometimes be challenging. When it comes to identifying skills and items for the résumé and the career portfolio, you'll want to use a combination of action verbs and keywords. The technology of today has shifted people's thinking—while they are still looking for action-oriented people (action verbs), they are also looking for ways to quickly dial into who and what you are by descriptive things you can do. What concrete terms can be used to describe you? Focus on the skills and keyword terms that are core to dietetics.

Add Keywords to Your Résumé

Keywords are terms that cue people into specific skills and abilities. If you've ever used a search engine on the Internet, you've used keywords. Think about your résumé as if it were a web site. What terms do you want people to look for and find? A person wanting to show her experience in project management might use keywords such as "coordinated," "grant," "$600,000," "solicited," "donations," and "outreach." Employers use keywords to screen applicants for interviews. Make sure your résumé makes the cut.

Action verbs are used on a résumé to describe what you have done. Here are a few action verbs to get you thinking:

accomplished, advised, assessed, authorized, budgeted, completed, conducted, demonstrated, managed, encouraged, maintained, recommended, scheduled, solved, etc.

A more extensive list of action verbs is included in chapter 9, "Resource Guide," for use in your résumé to indicate the action you have completed. Use them with keywords to demonstrate your skills. As a rule, scanned résumés look more at keywords, whereas a résumé reviewed by a person tends to note the action verbs. In the following descriptions the **action verb is in bold** and the keywords are underlined:

- **Managed** a team of four dietitians
- **Maintained** a database of 2,000 patients
- Meeting planning— Helped **plan, organize,** and **manage** the 2002, 2003, and 2004 New York State Annual Food and Nutrition Conference and Exposition — Committee member
- Webmaster — **designed** web site, **maintained** online registration, **managed** conference database and registration.

The Scannable Résumé

With the volume of applicants for positions, more companies are using computers to select potential candidates for the interview process. The software and scanning technology is quite advanced, and it is more cost effective than paying an employee to do the same work. With the thought in mind that your résumé may never be read by a real person, it's time to plan ahead and create a résumé that appeals to both the computer and the human reader. You can do this by using keywords and action verbs and by formatting the résumé in a way that can be scanned easily by a computer. Here are some guidelines for making your résumé scanner friendly:

- Use black ink on 8.5" x 11" white paper, printed only on one side.
- Don't use italic or underline.
- Use 12- to 14-pitch font size for body text and 16- to 18-pitch fonts for headings.
- Use a non-decorative type style.
- Place your name on each page in the header or footer.
- Use one-inch margins all the way around the document. (During the scanning process, margins are sometimes trimmed and information could be lost with a smaller margin.)
- Avoid using staples or folding the résumé on a line of text.
- Avoid the use of graphics, shading, and lines.
- Identify dates and times you are available at different contact addresses. Include e-mail addresses where possible.
- Use keywords—Using the vocabulary and terminology of dietetics is critical. Using terms like "trained teachers on recognizing and working with allergies," or "250 patients served," etc., may allow your résumé to be selected over another.

The following pages show a scannable résumé in the functional format:

Monique M. Derricote, MBA, RD

1234 West Way • Sacramento, CA 93233
(123) 456-7890 • mdd@provider.com

OBJECTIVE

I am seeking opportunities with a company that will allow me to utilize my management and health skills to promote health and nutrition.

EDUCATION

Masters of Business Administration – 2003   California State University; Sacramento, CA
- GPA: 3.40
- Relevant Courses: Accounting, Business Communications, Finance, Individual and Business Taxation, Management Information Systems, Marketing, Negotiations and Conflict, Operations Management, Research Methodology, Strategic Management
- Marketing Project: Developed a marketing plan to increase sales that was implemented by a local small business.

Dietetic Internship – 1999   Prairie View A&M University; Prairie View, TX
- Registered Dietitian -

Bachelors of Science: Dietetics; Food Technology Emphasis – 1998   Prairie View A&M University; Prairie View, TX
- GPA: 3.86 - Magna Cum Laude
- Benjamin Bannekar Honors College

SKILLS & QUALIFICATIONS

Project Management
- COORDINATED the implementation and administration of nutrition/physical education outreach grants totaling over $600,000
- OVERSAW and ADHERED to grant budgets
- EVALUATED the effectiveness of outreach programs and events; provided recommendations for improvement
- COLLABORATED with community and statewide organizations to develop and conduct health programs and events
- SOLICITED and OBTAINED financial and other donations worth over $10,000 from local and national agencies to enhance outreach efforts
- RECRUITED, TRAINED, and SUPERVISED staff, interns, and volunteers who assisted implementation of outreach events
- SUPERVISED one nutrition assistant and dietetic interns

Nutrition Education
- PLANNED, DEVELOPED, and CONDUCTED nutrition education classes for students, parents, teachers, and the community
- PARTICIPATED on community and national outreach panels and forums
- NETWORKED with medical and community organizations, parents, and teachers to enhance nutrition/physical education outreach program
- SURVEYED participants to determine nutrition/physical education needs
- TRAINED medical professionals, teachers, food service staff, parents, and the community on nutrition concepts
- EVALUATED skills acquired during trainings and conducted follow-ups with participants as needed

Marketing
- PLANNED, ORGANIZED, and ADMINISTERED health fairs, exhibit booths/boards, promotions, contests, programs, and presentations for grades K-12 and university students, parents, staff, and the community
- PARTICIPATED in television interviews and programs highlighting outreach efforts
- COORDINATED an annual field day event for over 750 participants
- INDEPENDENTLY DEVELOPED and PRESENTED brochures, biographical sheets, and PowerPoint presentations for the community and scientific, academic, and medical professionals
- IMPLEMENTED, DESIGNED, and EDITED monthly newsletters
- DISSEMINATED information about the accomplishments of the organization and its staff to stakeholders and for a federal report provided to the President of the United States
- UPDATED and MAINTAINED web sites

-Continued-

This professional résumé includes a summary of skills organized by area. It also integrates keywords and action verbs to describe work experiences.

WORK HISTORY

- *Consultant Dietitian*; Gentiva – Rehab Without Walls, Sacramento, CA, March 2003 - Present
- *Project Coordinator/Nutrition Educator*; Sacramento City Unified School District Nutrition Services, Sacramento, CA, December 2001 – Present
- *Certified Pump Trainer*; Medtronic MiniMed, Inc., Sacramento, CA, September 2001 – Present
- *Nutrition Information Coordinator*; USDA - Western Human Nutrition Research Center, Davis, CA, July 2000 – December 2001
- *Consultant Clinical Dietitian*; Doctors Medical Center, Modesto, CA, April 2000 – December 2001
- *Nutritionist*; USDA - Western Human Nutrition Research Center, Davis, CA, May 1999 – July 2000

ADDITIONAL SKILLS

Skills: Grant Writing • Press Releases • Media Relations • Newsletters
Software: Microsoft Office • Photoshop • PageMaker • FrontPage • NetObjects Fusion

PROFESSIONAL AFFILIATIONS

American Dietetic Association – New Member Advisory Committee Appointee 2002-2004; Chair 2004-2005 • American Diabetes Association – Volunteer • California Dietetic Association • Dietitians in Business and Communication Dietetic Practice Group • Golden Empire District Dietetic Association • National Organization of Blacks in Dietetics and Nutrition - Publicity Committee Chair 2001-2002 • Nutrition Entrepreneurs Dietetic Practice Group – 2005-2006 Newsletter Editor

Career Portfolio and References available for review

This professional résumé includes a summary of skills organized by area. It also integrates keywords and action verbs to describe work experiences.

Sending Out Your Résumé

Keep in mind your résumé is the tool that gets you an interview. Your résumé needs to represent you and should be a professional looking document. Be sure to double and triple check your résumé for typos, formatting errors, and correct information. Simple errors can show a lack of attention to details and may cause your résumé to be automatically rejected by some employers.

Cover Letters

A cover letter is sent with the résumé and should briefly explain what sets you apart from others and why you would be the best person for the job. Employers use the cover letter to check for writing style, attention to detail and tone, as well as your qualifications. Here are a few "do's" for cover letters:

- Check your spelling and grammar
- Address the letter to the specific person who will be reviewing your letter
- Draw attention to key summaries of your résumé
- Explain what types of opportunities you are looking to secure.

E-Mailing Your Résumé

Occasionally you may be asked to e-mail your résumé to a prospective employer or contact at an organization. This is often the case when you have a personal contact with someone in the organization. E-mailing your résumé gives you quick-strike ability. You can react faster and have your résumé on the employer's desk faster than with regular mail. Here are some general guidelines to follow when e-mailing a résumé:

- **Send your résumé as an attachment—** Send the résumé as a Word file or an Adobe PDF (Portable Document File) so it can be printed out by the receiver.
- **Include a cover letter—** Send the cover letter as an attachment, or write your cover letter in the body of the e-mail.

- **Include your contact information in the body of the e-mail—** This way if there are any problems with the files, the receiver can get to you as quickly as possible.

- **Use standard fonts like Times New Roman or Arial when sending your résumé document—** If the receiver's computer doesn't have your funky font installed, your document will print with different fonts and will not look its best.

- **Save your résumé in a PDF format if possible—** You need to have Adobe Acrobat on your computer to create a PDF. The recipient must have a program called Acrobat Viewer on their computer. The Viewer can be downloaded from the Internet for free. This format can be printed directly from a browser screen. The PDF files cannot be edited or changed by anyone else, and your fonts and formatting will be intact.

- **Use your private e-mail, not a corporate account—** Organizations have the right to monitor their employees' e-mail. If you are currently employed and looking for another job, you should correspond through a private e-mail account, not the corporate address. You probably don't want your current employer to know you're actively looking for a new job.

- **Send a hard copy of your résumé and cover letter by mail—** Follow up your e-mail with a hard copy to reinforce your e-mail message and to serve as a backup copy.

Faxing Your Résumé

You can also respond quickly to a request by faxing your résumé to an employer. Since the quality of a fax machine copy is inferior to a printed hard copy, you should send this only at the request of the organization. Here are a few guidelines to consider when faxing a résumé:

- **Fax from a copy of your résumé printed on white paper—** Colored paper and paper with texture do not fax well and tend to be grainy and hard to read. White paper will fax better.

- **Include a cover letter—** Send the cover letter and résumé together with a cover sheet directed to the correct person.

- **Use standard fonts like Times New Roman or Arial when sending your résumé**— Again, funky fonts don't always print well on the other end of the fax machine.

- **Consider the uses of your office fax machine**— The sending fax machine produces a log of all faxes sent. It often lists the name of the organization at the receiving end of a fax. Consider carefully if you want your employer to know you're faxing things to another organization or competitor. Many copy shops and mail centers offer faxing services.

- **Make sure the fax goes through**— Be sure you stand at the machine until the fax has been successfully sent. If it doesn't go through or the line is busy it may drop your fax job. Wait for a confirmation statement from the fax machine.

- **Send a hard copy of your résumé and cover letter by mail**— Follow up your fax with a hard copy to reinforce your message and to serve as a backup copy.

New Trends in Résumés

Online Résumé Services

These days you may find your job by placing your résumé in an electronic database. A growing number of services will scan your résumé and place it on the Internet or other database services. Many of these web sites are geared to people in certain industries. Such sites are popular with employers because they can get the résumés of prospective employees who are already screened to a certain industry.

Some services will scan your résumé and ask you to complete a brief application, including items such as salary preferences, employers, willingness to travel, distance willing to travel, etc. The service gives employers access to "at-a-glance" peeks at your résumé. For a fee, they will give an employer a copy of the entire résumé via fax. After that, it's up to the employer to contact you.

Some of these services will provide you with feedback on who requested your résumé and the salary ranges other professionals with similar skills are earning in the industry. They will also identify trends in professional fields, such as a need for increased computer skills in nutritional analysis software.

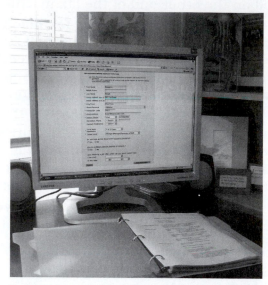

Online résumés are becoming commonplace.

Professional databases are available not only to college graduates, but also to professionals trying to determine the marketability of their skills. You can find these databases by browsing on the Internet using key terms such as **career placement**, **job search**, and **employment**. Within the databases, you can search for openings by experience, salary ranges, key interest areas, etc. For using these services you will sometimes pay a flat fee of $25 to $75. In other cases, your résumé is scanned for free and the employer pays for access.

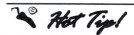

Recruiters at today's job fairs may ask you to upload your résumé to a web site or provide it electronically.

College Placement Web Sites

Many colleges and university placement centers have embraced the Internet and are using it to the advantage of graduates and alumni alike. Many schools keep a résumé database, whereas others are providing students with space for personal web pages. If you have the opportunity to create your own web site, check out Chapter 6, The Electronic Portfolio, for tips and guidelines for creating your site.

Web Page Résumés

More people are now putting résumés online with their own web pages. The really savvy people are creating more than just résumés—they're creating online portfolios. It's especially critical your résumé be well developed so you can gain the attention of the person searching your page. Links and key terms are critical. See chapter 6, "The Electronic Portfolio," for more details.

Writing a Brief Biography

A brief biography is often required in the dietetics field. It is a short summary of your qualities and qualifications. It usually contains an overview of your education, work experiences, memberships, community service activities, and your professional interests. A bio is often used when working with the media or when giving presentations. In your portfolio, the brief bio is placed in front of your résumé.

When writing your brief bio, you want to be sure to make it pleasant and conversational. Try to make it interesting and not a boring list of everything you can do. As with your résumé, you want to carefully pick which items to include in your bio. Your bio should have a mix of current and past achievements. Include relevant professional memberships, leadership roles, and volunteerism experiences. You want your bio to be professional, but you may include a personal description of your family or interests at the end.

It can sometimes be hard to list your accomplishments and still be humble about it. Try to imagine it being read out loud to someone. Does it give a person insight into who you are and what experiences you have to offer?

Here is a sample brief bio:

MARTIN M. YADRICK, MS, MBA, RD, FADA

Marty Yadrick is a member of the ADA Board of Directors and serves on the House of Delegates Leadership Team. He was recently elected ADA Treasurer-Elect and will begin his term on June 1, 2004. He was chair of ADA's Diversity Committee in 2001-2002, and is a past spokesperson for the association. Marty has served on the boards of both the California and Missouri Dietetic Associations. He was chair of the SCAN Dietetic Practice Group in 1993-94.

Mr. Yadrick is marketing manager for Computrition, Inc., a California-based provider of software solutions to the hospitality and health-care industries. Prior to moving to the Los Angeles area in 1993, he was administrative officer for the Department of Dietetics & Nutrition at the University of Kansas Medical Center.

Marty received his Bachelor of Science degree from Colorado State University, a Master of Science from the University of Kansas Medical Center, and a Master of Business Administration from the University of Missouri-Kansas City. He is a Fellow of the American Dietetic Association and is a past Recognized Young Dietitian of the Year recipient from Missouri. Marty also received the 2001 Excellence in Private Practice, Business, or Communications Award from the California Dietetic Association and the 2004 Achievement Award from the SCAN DPG.

Your Résumé Sets the Stage

In chapter 2 you planned out your portfolio and decided where to focus your efforts. By developing your résumé, you have identified the educational and job-related experiences you want to emphasize. You have really created an overview of your portfolio, the first step to creating the finished product. Use your résumé as a guide in the next two chapters as you begin to collect and organize work samples. As you begin to sort and decide on work samples, you may find your résumé needs to be adjusted. Congratulations! You're on your way to creating a focused portfolio that will help provide backup and support to your résumé!

Related Web Sites

Here are just a few of the thousands of web sites designed to help you create the perfect résumé. Use these sites as guidelines. Remember, you are creating a product that represents **you** to potential employers. Follow your instincts and create the résumé that feels right to you.

- **Career Builder** - http://www.careerbuilder.com
- **Chronicle of Higher Education** - http://chronicle.com/jobs/
- **Exercise Jobs** - http://www.exercisejobs.com/jobs/jobs_search.html
- **Health Careers** - http://www.healthcareers.com/
- **HotJobs @ Yahoo** - http://hotjobs.yahoo.com/
- **Idealist Community Nutrition** - http://www.idealist.org/
- **Nutrition Jobs** - http://www.nutritionjobs.com/
- **America's Job Bank** - http://www.ajb.dni.us/
- **CareerCity** - http://www.careercity.com/
- **CareerMagazine** - http://www.careermag.com/
- **CareerWeb** - http://www.careerweb.com/
- **JobBank USA** - Jobs MetaSEARCH - http://www.jobbankusa.com/search.html/
- **JobTrak** - http://www.jobtrak.com/
- **Resumail** - http://www.resumail.com/
- **ResumeBlaster** - http://www.resumeblaster.com/
- **The Job Hunters Bible** - *What Color Is My Parachute?* - http://www.jobhuntersbible.com/
- **The Monster Board** - http://www.monster.com/

- **Weddle's Web Guide** - http://www.nbew.com/
- **The Career Clinic** - http://www.thecareerclinic.com/

 Taking Action!

- Evaluate your employment and education. Determine what keywords and action verbs to use in your résumé.
- Develop your résumé.
- Write up your brief biography.

CHAPTER 4

PROVING YOUR SKILLS

This chapter is all about proof. Chapters 2 and 3 helped determine what skill areas you need to emphasize. Now we'll take that information and look at how to find, create, and select work samples, certificates, letters of recommendation, skill sets, and support materials which make up the heart of your portfolio. In this chapter you'll find the details on:

- Finding and choosing work samples
- Asking for and using letters of recommendation
- Creating works in progress
- Working with skill sets
- Using certifications, diplomas, degrees, and awards
- Using community service to prove your skills
- Using academic plan of study and faculty/employer bios
- Creating the reference materials needed to support your portfolio.

Look at the Big Picture

Take a look at your own skills and decide what areas you want to emphasize in your portfolio. Some possible areas include:

- Communications
- Management
- Clinical or community nutrition
- Marketing and public relations
- Research
- Government
- Private practice
- Food service management
- Wellness/fitness
- Sports nutrition

- Academia
- Extended care/assisted living
- Publications
- Teaching
- Training.

Try to choose three to five different areas that relate to you. Then select work samples that correspond to these areas. If you don't have very many work samples, you may find yourself creating categories to support your samples. It's important to make sure the samples you use support your goals and will show your best work.

Work Samples

Work samples make up the major portion of the portfolio and become the most powerful part of your sales pitch.

Work samples are proof of your knowledge and skills. When assembling your portfolio for an interview, you can customize your work samples to match the skills needed for the position. You can "wow" a potential employer by showing examples that clearly demonstrate skills he or she wants to see. Work samples also add to your credibility. Instead of just telling someone what you have done, you can show examples.

Sources of Work Samples

Common sources for work samples include:

- Classroom projects from your dietetics courses during school
- Materials you have generated while on the job or in your internship
- Materials completed in community service projects or professional memberships.

Class Assignments

Projects you developed to fulfill course requirements are a great source of work samples. The grade you earned on the project is usually not included, but could be brought up as a point of discussion in the interview. Some examples include:

- Real-life simulations
- A feasibility study you generated in a marketing class
- The menu you created for your menu design project or capstone food course
- A business plan you developed
- An advertising campaign you developed as a team effort
- Office or facility designs.

Anything you create that shows your skill in a particular area can be used as a work sample. If the physical evidence is too big to fit in the portfolio (like a poster or diagram), take a picture of the item and include the photo.

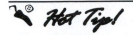

Use a photo when a large 3-D project doesn't fit into your career portfolio.

Try to find samples that are interesting. You may have a great report you did for a class, but 15 pages of double-spaced text is boring. Creating a one-page overview that highlights what you covered and what you learned can be a better sample to include in the portfolio.

The more details you can give about the project, the better. You may want to include some of the following items for each project sample:

- The project assignment sheet— you may have to rekey it so that it is presentable
- Table of contents for the entire project
- Names of people working on the project
- Assignment summaries
- Why it was generated, the purpose it served
- Executive summaries if possible
- Financial summaries where appropriate
- Pictures
- Multimedia summaries
- What you learned from the project
- Any prerequisites to this assignment.

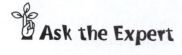

Ask the Expert

I got rid of all my projects . . .

Q. I have done lots of class projects, but have lost or thrown most of them away. What can I put in my portfolio to show my experiences?

A. It's always frustrating when you realize you had great class projects that would show experience but you've cleared your "clutter" and thrown them away. If you are still in school, check and see if your instructor has an assignment sheet for the project, which could be included in the portfolio. You could also write up a project summary. List the assignment, what you created, and what you learned from it. Keep the project summary sheet to a single page. Depending on the type of project, you may also have photos that could be used.

On-the-Job Samples, Co-Op Projects, or Internship Projects

Having a hard time coming up with work samples? Take a look at the things you do on the job and consider the things you create and work with on a daily basis that show your experience. Take a look at chapter 9, "Resource Guide," for work sample ideas. Consider using some of these work samples:

- Departmental operating procedures
- Programs or systems you have created
- Article you wrote for the local newspaper
- Market research techniques
- Promotional materials
- Job projects such as employee newsletters
- Special events created
- Multimedia presentations created
- Purchasing forms used
- Budgets developed
- Overview of proposals and grants written
- Photos of yourself in action
- Forms you have created to assist staff.

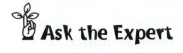

Ask the Expert

I need some experience!

Q. I recently obtained my diploma and graduated with honors, but in my field there aren't many jobs open. Those that are advertising want someone with experience. So far, I have my résumé posted on several job search web sites, but that hasn't been too productive. Any advice?

A. It seems you have a lot to offer. There are a couple of ways to address the work experience problem:

1. Seek out a paid internship with a respected company. Go in with an educational contract where you want to have specific work experience to document. You need at least six months' experience and often this can be worked around another position as long as you are up front as to what you want to accomplish.

2. Find any class projects you generated which could serve as work samples in your career portfolio.

3. You need to be prepared for more than just the obvious fields where you can use your skills. Determine your transferable skills and find out other industries that need people with these skills. Broaden your search. Join a professional association where you can network and become known—it adds to your credibility while you build work experience.

Community Service Projects

Community involvement is a great source of work samples often overlooked by people as they pull together their portfolios. Service samples may be written projects or pictures of your involvement in community service. Examples include:

- The PowerPoint slides from the "Healthy Dieting" presentation you gave to the local women's group
- The grant proposal you helped create for a day-care facility
- A flyer you created for the June newsletter
- A picture of your team feeding residents in a long-term care facility

- A photo of you working in a soup kitchen
- The menu you developed for the PTA dinner
- The menu and production plan for a catered dinner for 80.

Include the following information for each community service sample:

- A summary sheet of what you accomplished
- Results of the project
- Who helped you
- A photo if appropriate.

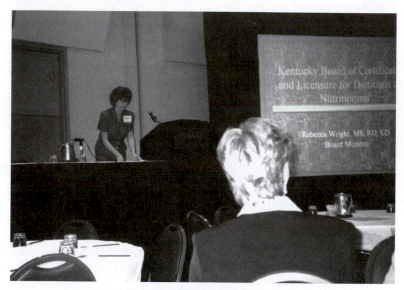

Photos of yourself in action are a great way
to show your community service.

If your community service samples relate to one of your skill areas, you may choose to put your sample there. If your service experience doesn't relate, you should create a separate tabbed section for community service.

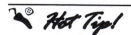

Employers like to see community service involvement. Use your volunteerism to demonstrate your skills.

Your Commitment to Personal Growth

Employers want to know you are committed to the job and to the company. They also want to see you grow and expand professionally because it's good for business. Having a plan for your own professional development and growth in your field shows your commitment to yourself and the field of dietetics. Most people achieve professional growth through professional memberships and certifications.

Professional Memberships and Services

Professional memberships and services show your commitment to the field and demonstrate how you will keep up with the growing and changing knowledge/skills in the field. You should be carrying at least one professional membership at all times. What professional groups should you belong to? Here's a sampling of professional groups to choose from:

- American Dietetic Association (ADA) and its Dietetic Practice Groups (DPGs)
- American Society for Parenteral and Enteral Nutrition (ASPEN)
- American Society for Nutritional Sciences (ASNS)
- American Society for Clinical Nutrition (ASCN)
- National Restaurant Association (NRA)
- American Society of Hospital Food Service Administrators (ASHFSA)
- American Hospital Association (AHA)
- The Wellness Council of America
- American Diabetes Association.

Seeking out leadership roles in a professional organization is one way to demonstrate your management and leadership abilities.

Professional memberships are usually listed under a separate tabbed area in your portfolio and are usually no more than two to four pages in length. You should include the following information:

- A list of organizations to which you belong.

- The date you joined.
- Offices, boards, or committees on which you've served.
- Appropriate letters of accomplishment.
- Photographs of events or copies of programs where you have provided a presentation or service.
- Provide proof of your membership. Use a membership card or a letter from the president of the organization as proof of your membership. If your membership card is your canceled check, use the letter instead.
- Spell out the name of the organization, don't just use its abbreviation. Listing a membership in the ADA could be referring to the American Dental Association, American Diabetes Association or the American Dietetic Association.

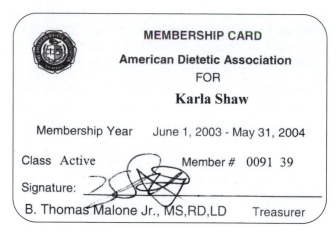

Professional memberships show your desire to grow in your career.

Sample:

Professional Memberships

- American Dietetic Association (ADA)— Member since 2002
    - ♦ Nominating Committee— 2004–Present
- Kappa Omicron Nu, The National Honor Society in Family and Consumer Sciences, since 2002.

Template

Use the template on the enclosed disk to create your own membership listing. **(Memberships.doc)**

Using the Portfolio to Track Certifications and Professional Development

As we said in the first chapter, a portfolio is a great tool for managing information. The portfolio is the perfect place to store all your certificates, checklists, and plans.

Be sure to collect work samples as you complete your continuing education. Projects, letters of recommendation, and skill sets help document your experience. If you are in the process of completing a certification in a specific area, make sure one of your career goals is the completion of the certification program.

Keep in mind that certifications and advanced degrees can take a considerable amount of time and effort to complete. Ask yourself some of these questions to determine why you want the degree:

- Does your future career path require a certificate or degree to be qualified?
- Will your salary increase enough to pay for the cost of advanced education over time?
- Do you enjoy learning? Advanced degrees can be more interesting than undergraduate work because they focus on a particular area, but they often require great amounts of timely work.

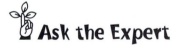 **Ask the Expert**

Do I need certification?

Q. Do I need certifications after I become a RD?

A. Some RDs hold additional certifications in specialized areas of practice, such as pediatric nutrition (Board Certified Specialist in Pediatric Nutrition), renal nutrition (Board Certified Specialist in Renal Nutrition), nutrition support (Board Certified Nutrition Support Dietitian), and diabetes education (Board Certified Diabetes Educator). Some of these certifications are awarded through CDR, the credentialing agency for ADA, and others are awarded by credible organizations recognized within the profession such as the National Board of Nutrition Support Certification or the National Certification Board for Diabetes Educators. Certifications are not required but some employers do prefer higher certified people. You are required to complete continuing professional educational requirements to maintain your registration.

Certificates from short term training programs such as weight management (Certificate of Training in Adult Weight Management Program and the Certificate of Training in Childhood and Adolescent Weight Management) can also be used to prove your skills, but do not include the same intense training and testing as certification programs.

Memberships and certifications can help prove to an employer that you are serious about your job and your career. Take some time to look at your master plan and decide how this can all work together to advance your career. Education is valued, and when packaged correctly, you can open many doors and have fun.

Managing Your Work Samples

Work samples are the dynamic portion of your portfolio. As you prepare for different job interviews, your portfolio needs to be adjusted as well. You may need to change the work samples you show to demonstrate specific abilities that are desired by the company. You need to evaluate your portfolio before each interview to make sure it fits the prospective employer's needs. Selecting the correct work samples and keeping them organized for instant access is very important. Follow these guidelines to help you choose your samples:

- **How to select the best work samples—** Ask yourself the following questions about each sample:
  - What will this work demonstrate—skills, competencies, or achievement of goals?
  - Is this my best work?
  - Does it show mastery?

- ♦ Am I proud of this sample . . . all or part of it?
- **Include a sample, not the whole project**— Try to limit yourself to a maximum of 5-7 pages per project. People don't want to read everything.
- **Offer the full project**— Add a line on a work sample overview card offering the full project:

Full project available upon request

- **Identify people who contributed to the project**— When presenting work samples, clearly identify its purpose and everyone who has contributed to the sample.
- **When in doubt, leave it out**— Never include a work sample that you are not proud to be associated with, now or in the future. Remember more is not necessarily better.
- **Use a photo summary**— A photo summary of your work may be the best way to relay a work experience. Create photos which show summaries of your work, not just the physical environment. Include pictures of yourself in action with the project.
- **Make it look good**— Select the best way to present your work samples: through text or photos. (See chapter 8, "A Matter of Style," for more information.)
- **Use grouped sheet protectors for projects**— You can purchase special sets of five or 10 interconnected sheet protectors. Use these to keep an entire project sample together so you can easily switch out projects in the portfolio when customizing it to the employer.
- **Pay attention to confidentiality**— Materials generated on the job are usually the property of the company you were working for at the time you created the material. When you display or show that material, be sure to recognize the owner. If you have signed a confidentiality agreement with a company, you should not include their work in your portfolio.

It's Confidential . . .

John included materials from his job in his work samples and indicated on the sample cards the material was used with permission. He interviewed with his portfolio but didn't get the job. When he asked the interviewer for feedback, the interviewer said he was concerned about how an applicant who used confidential samples in an interview would handle confidentiality on the job.

Keeping Track of Your Work Samples

- **Have a schedule for updating your collection of work samples**— Develop a routine for collecting materials. If you are in school, you may choose midterm and final exam time to stop and consider which, if any, of your projects should be saved for your files. On the job, make a 30- to 60-minute appointment with yourself once every quarter to take time to reflect on your work over the past months. You should consider completed reports, projects, awards, achievements, or project summaries.

- **Keep track of your work samples**— Get a large plastic tote with folders. You should keep original copies of projects, letters of recommendations, letters of accommodation, or certificates of achievement or degrees. You don't need to spend lots of time arranging it; you just need a designated place to keep your materials.

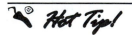 *Hot Tip!*

Documents with some color show better than plain black and white. Use color copies or printouts if possible.

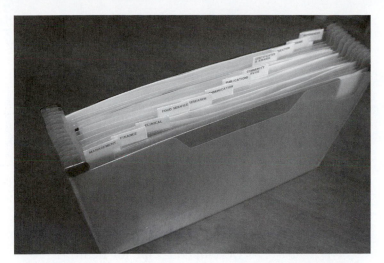

Use a file to store your work samples and supplies.

- **Include the correct work samples—** The work samples you include in your portfolio will vary, based on the needs of the potential employer. You should have a collection of different work samples stored in your tote or filing cabinet. Each sample should be in its own set of sheet protectors, so you can quickly swap out appropriate work samples as needed.

- **Organize work samples into the appropriate skill areas—** Work samples should be clustered by major skill areas. You determine these skill areas. Each skill area will have its own tabbed section in the portfolio. Each skill area should contain work samples that emphasize that particular area.

- **Organize work samples within a skill area—** The organization and flow of work samples will vary with each sample. Try to break up text and photos so the arrangement creates growing interest and piques curiosity. You may want to organize your work samples in a flow that shows your growth or chronological advancement.

- **Use overview cards for each sample—** An overview card is a small card containing a brief summary of the work sample. It is placed inside the page protector of the first page of your sample and helps the reader remember what he or she is looking at and why. We recommend you create cards for each work sample using a blank sheet of standard size business cards. Format the page on your computer, and include the following information:

- ◆ Title of the sample
- ◆ Purpose of the sample
- ◆ Date of work
- ◆ Who worked with you (if anyone)
- ◆ What skills are demonstrated using keywords.

Recipe for a Healthy Heart

Prime Life Magazine, Spring 2005

Developed recipe for health-conscious individuals

Skills: Knowledge of low-calorie, low-fat diet; writing ability, creativity

---

Create an overview card for each sample in your portfolio.

 Template

Use the template on the enclosed disk to create your own overview cards. **(Work Sample Overview Cards.doc)**

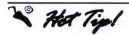

Check your samples for abbreviations. Don't assume people will know what they mean. See the list of Common Dietetics Professional Abbreviations in chapter 9, "Resource Guide."

Letters of Recommendation

Letters of recommendation from employers, instructors, etc., can provide additional proof of your abilities. Letters provide personal references from people who have seen you perform. You may need to rely more on letters of recommendation when you don't have many work samples, or when the type of work you do doesn't facilitate written samples.

You should ask for letters from people who know you and/or your work personally. Instructors, supervisors, owners, presidents, and managers—all can be appropriate references. Whoever you choose should be familiar with your work and be able to judge performance and competency. You should be proud to be associated with these people. If you don't like them, they probably don't like you, and you don't want a letter from them.

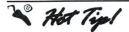 *Hot Tip!*

Use letters of recommendation in your portfolio when you don't have a lot of physical work samples.

Asking for a Letter

- You should request your letter of recommendation in writing long before you need it. If you are in school, ask your teacher for the recommendation soon after taking his or her class.

- Your letter needs to help guide the person writing the recommendation to focus his or her letter on key skills and areas of your personality that you want addressed.

- Ask for the letter while you are close to the event or you still have an opportunity for contact with the person.

- You should always allow two to three weeks for receiving the letter, as people tend to get busy. It is appropriate to follow up with them a week after your request. Don't be afraid to proof their work. If you find a mistake, be humble and ask for a correction.

To ask for a recommendation, remember to start with courtesy and manners; say please and thank you frequently, and in a heartfelt way. Remember, these people hold your success in the palm of their hands. Your goal, the purpose of a letter, is to document your performance, to have your achievement recognized, and/or to have your abilities summarized. **Most people write lousy letters of recommendation.** They tend to make the letters too general or generic. You need to help the person you choose to write the letter. When writing your letter, begin by telling the person the purpose of the letter: for your portfolio, for graduate school, for an internship, or a press release. Then, dial in your reference by giving them a list of traits, skills, or attributes you want addressed. Here are some examples:

- Leadership
- Ability to work in groups
- Ability to self-motivate
- Ability to meet customer needs
- Ability to complete work
- Ability to supervise

- Management skills
- Creativity
- People skills
- Bilingual
- Specialized skills you possess (speciality in pediatrics, sports nutrition, etc.).

The Perfect Letter

The letter should be on official letterhead, should have an ink signature, and should not be folded. The recommendation letter you receive should be addressed as "Dear Future Employer." Do not use the generic, open-ended salutations such as "To Whom It May Concern" . . . or "Dear Sir or Madame." It should also include background information on how the reference knows you and how long you have been associated with the organization or project. He or she should explain how long you have been associated and in what capacity.

Letters of recommendation will go in one of three places in the portfolio—work sample documentation, professional service/membership, and/or community service. If the letter is comprehensive, discussing two or more of these sections, include it in the work samples and refer to it in the other area. A sample request letter is shown on the next page.

 Template

A sample recommendation request letter is included on the accompanying diskette. Use it as a starting point for writing your own letters. **(Recommendation request.doc)**

Sample Request Letter

Inside Address

Today's date

Dear Professor Watkins:

I was a student of yours last term in your Advanced Medical Nutrition Therapy class. I earned an A in your class, and was an active participant every day so you probably remember me. I will be graduating in May, and I am currently working on assembling my career portfolio. Could you please write a letter of recommendation addressing the following skills:

- My ability to work in teams
- My ability to present findings professionally
- My ability to identify diet-related health problems
- My ability to recommend nutrient intakes.

It would also be helpful if you could indicate how long you have known me and on what occasions you have worked with me. I would appreciate it if you could address the letter to "Dear Future Employer" and leave the letter unfolded.

I would greatly appreciate receiving this letter within the next two weeks. Please call or e-mail me and let me know when it would be convenient for me to pick up the letter. Thank you very much for your consideration and all your help. Please feel free to call me if you have any questions.

Sincerely,

Russell Jackson

Russell Jackson

123 45th Ave.

Any State, NY 01011

(123) 456-7890 - Home phone

e-mail: rsljksn@provider.com

Here's the letter received in response to the request.

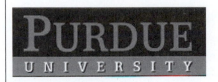

Marcus Watkins, Ph.D.
Purdue University
7777 Main Street
West Lafayette, IN 47906

May 14, 2004

Dear Future Employer:

I am pleased to write this letter of recommendation for Russell Jackson. I had the opportunity to teach Russell in my Advanced Medical Nutritional Therapy class. He stood out as an exemplary student.

Russell has many valuable qualities. Very goal-oriented, Russell was always punctual, yet easygoing. He was keenly devoted to his course work, but being a real people person, he was also enjoyable to be around.

Russell completed several course projects during the class, many of which required group interaction. His ability to work with groups, as well as his leadership skills, were obvious. Russell was extremely comfortable in presenting his research and findings from his assignments orally to the class. He was clear, precise, and always prepared for questions.

The class required much research, as well as hands-on work. Russell excelled in both areas. Some of the skills Russell was able to develop in my class included identifying diet-related health problems, recommending nutrient level intakes, and counseling skills. After completing the course-work, I feel that Russell can perform these skills with ease.

In closing, let me say I have no hesitation in recommending Russell Jackson for any supervisory position in dietetics. I feel confident he would be an asset to your organization.

Sincerely,

Marcus C. Watkins

Professor, Food Science Department

Ask the Expert

Using nonacademic activities

Q. I am involved in a lot of nonacademic activities. Is there anything I should use in my career portfolio?

A. Yes. Employers respect transferable skills, especially in the area of soft skills or interpersonal skills such as teamwork, presentation skills, leadership, problem solving, and others. Good ways to document these skills are through:

- Letters of referral
- Customer comment letters
- Awards and recognitions received.

Be sure to link the skills you gain from nonacademic activities to the position you are targeting. Use your project overview cards to link the work sample to the skill sets you are trying to demonstrate. Sports, clubs, and especially community service can all serve as excellent sources of skill development. Be sure to collect your work samples now—you can sort them later as you customize your portfolio to your targeted employer.

Works in Progress

This is a place to list projects on which you are currently working. You may choose to show parts or modules that are completed enough to demonstrate a skill, competency, or achievement. This section may be very short. It should be clearly labeled "Works in Progress," and can be placed at the beginning of the work samples in an area. You may want to use a bulleted list. During an interview, you may refer to this list of current projects after you have discussed your work samples. It can serve to transition the interviewer or supervisor into more questions. Your list should include:

- The expected completion date
- Whom the work is for
- What skills or competencies it demonstrates.

Skill Sets

What Are Skill Sets?

So, what if you just do not have a lot of physical work samples available? A listing of your skills and how well you can perform them can be used in your portfolio to demonstrate your skills and abilities. A **skill set** is a list of related skills that are grouped together. Skill competencies from your dietetic internship rotations are excellent samples to include in your portfolio. Each set is signed off on by the internship director or preceptor.

Skill sets are not only a list of your abilities, but they also show the level of your abilities. Skills and competencies should be graded by ability. Many skill sets will work with each skill or competency, using three levels of ability:

Awareness— Has awareness of the knowledge/skill, and has completed the task at least once.

Practicing— Is able to follow a guide to complete a task.

Mastery— Is able to consistently perform the task without effort.

The following pages show a skill set created to track competencies in food handling and preparation.

Food Handling and Preparation

Awareness	Practicing	Mastery
Has awareness of the knowledge/skill, and/or has completed the task at least once.	Is able to follow a guide to complete the task.	Is able to consistently perform the task without effort.

Is able to develop a low-sodium diet.

print name	print name	print name
signature	signature	signature
date	date	date

Is able to establish a specialized patient diet.

print name	print name	print name
signature	signature	signature
date	date	date

Is able to handle and prepare food safely.

print name	print name	print name
signature	signature	signature
date	date	date

Is able to communicate the importance of following dietary guidelines.

print name	print name	print name
signature	signature	signature
date	date	date

Is able to update dietary cardex.

print name	print name	print name
signature	signature	signature
date	date	date

Is able to prepare and update tray cards.

print name	print name	print name
signature	signature	signature
date	date	date

Is able to ensure food quality.

print name	print name	print name
signature	signature	signature
date	date	date

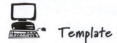 Template

A blank skill set is included on the accompanying diskette. Use it as a starting point for creating your own skill sets. **(Skillset.doc)**

The style of the skill set shown allows you to track your progress on achieving your goals and increasing your skill levels. This skill set features space for a credible professional or educator to sign off on your level of ability. It is important you take responsibility for getting your skills measured and signed off on. This is especially critical if you do not have a lot of work samples to support those skills.

Think ahead! It is always more difficult to get a signature after the employment or class is over, since the person being asked to sign off may not have as clear a memory of your work. Additionally, be sure to request biographical information at the time you receive the signature so you can include the information on a Faculty and Employer Biography sheet.

Creating Your Own Skill Sets

It is not difficult to make your own skill sets and use them to prove your abilities. To create your own skill sets:

■ **Use job descriptions to identify skills you want to have—** Not all job descriptions are well written; however, there are usually key abilities identified in the text. Shop through the job requirements and evaluate your skills against the requirements, looking for terminology. In fact, a really great way to evaluate your own skills is to write the job description for your ideal position and then check if you meet the qualifications. The Career Development office at your local community college, university, or professional association may be of some assistance if you are not quite sure where to look for job descriptions. You can also find many job descriptions online. Check the web sites listed at the end of Chapter 3, "The Resume," for additional resources.

■ **Use job ads or job postings to identify and check skills—** Check the Sunday papers for job advertisements. Look in *Today's Dietitian*, *JADA*, or Nutritionjobs.com to find job postings. Look at the requirements of the ad and the keywords used to identify the skills needed for the position. Look at the skills, written and implied.

Now expand and refine this list of skills . . .

- **List the things you have done on the job—** Reflect on your own life and work experiences. List all the things you do in the course of a day . . . week . . . month. This usually covers your routine skills. Break your time down so you can clearly think through the entire period of time. Try to be very specific; rather than saying, "as a supervisor I work with people to prepare food for the patients," consider also your responsibility for sanitation, flow of the tray line, and ensuring the proper procedures are followed. Can you do each person's job if asked? Many times we underestimate all the skills and tasks we do in a day.

- **List unique skills—** Things special to the position, those things you get asked to do because you are better at it than others. Focus on your patient education skills, your problem-solving skills, or your ability to manage a tray line.

- **List your transferable skills—** Those that can be used in many different positions. Consider the skills you have that are not necessarily specific to dietetics, skills you may have obtained in other areas of your life. If you are weak in certain skill areas such as leadership or planning, seek out community service opportunities to enhance those skills.

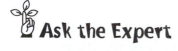 **Ask the Expert**

No physical samples of my work!

Q. What do I do if I don't have any good work samples? I haven't kept many of my work samples, and I'm not sure what to do now.

A. Start by exploring the skills you have. Make a list of all the skills you know you have. Then target people who can help you document your skills. Consider teachers, employers, and even personal references that hold good standing. Ask them to write you a letter of reference or participation. Take the time to guide them by letting them know exactly what skills you want them to address in their letters.

Another way to document your skills is by using a skill set. A skill set is a list of skills that have been grouped together. Make a list of your skill sets and ask your employers or instructors to sign off verifying your skills. It is best to use a combination of employers and instructors to help document your skills.

Get A Head Start . . .
Create Your Skill Sets in School or on the Job

Customize your skill sets based on your course work—
While you are in school or still in a learning setting, take time at the beginning of each term or rotation to review the skills and competencies you expect to secure, refine, or learn. Once you've completed the course, you should be able to identify new skills and at what level you can perform the skills; awareness, practicing, or mastery levels.

Imagine going into a class or internship rotation knowing what you want to get out of it and then working with the instructor to create your own learning plan. You want to be proactive rather than reactive to your education. This keeps you from being a "passive user" of the educational system. (Remember to keep good work samples for possible use later.)

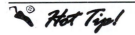 *Hot Tip!*

You are responsible for your own education! Go into a class or internship rotation knowing what you want to get out of it and work to create your own learning plan. Be proactive rather than reactive to your education!

Professionals on the job—At the beginning of a job or review period, you should clearly decide what skills you have, need, or want to prove, and which ones you want to develop during the next year. You need to give yourself enough structure so you can grow within the company and as a professional in dietetics. Consider incorporating your skill needs into your performance goals for the year. This is a good way to strategically organize yourself, especially if you make sure your goals and the company's goals interface or map back to each other.

Certifications, Diplomas, Registration Status, Degrees, or Awards

Remember, you need to prove the things you have done. Professional certificates related to areas of specialty, such as Certified Diabetes Educator, ADA leadership training certification, continuing education, workshops attended, distinctions, or commendations are appropriate items to place in your portfolio. Here are some tips for using certificates and awards:

- **Include a copy of the certificate—** Include a quality photocopy or scanned image of the certificate or diploma as proof and verification. Don't include the original.

- **Include information about the organization presenting the certificate—** The certificate should be dated and have information about the organization. If it does not, add the following items to your overview card:
  - ◆ Name
  - ◆ Address and phone number of the organization
  - ◆ Any certification or licensing numbers given.

- **Place the most recent items first—** If you have any citations (not speeding or parking tickets!) for service, include them with the most current items first. For example, if you received the customer service award at work last year, and you received dean's list this term—place the dean's list before the customer service award.

- **Be selective—** What goes in here? Everything? No. Show items that will be of interest to your future employer. Do your homework on the interests of the organization with which you are applying or currently working for today. Remember more is not necessarily better.

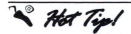

Use color copies of originals and keep the original in a safe place. NEVER put the original copy of a project or certificate in your portfolio!

Community Service

There ARE Other Ways to Get Experience

Being an active volunteer is very important in the dietetics field. Many education programs require community service as a component of education. Your volunteer experience is a required section of the Dietetic Internship Application, with both dietetic and non-dietetic experience desired.

People who are not actively in the work force or those people who have been out for a while can use their volunteer projects as a way to demonstrate skills and secure proof, without having held employment. If you are looking for experience, go to an organization and offer your services free of charge. Start a project and see it through to the end. Be sure to make it clear that all you want is a letter documenting your time and skills. Then have some fun and test drive, develop, or refine your skills.

Great Volunteer Opportunities Here!

- Cooperative extensions
- Health centers
- Meals on Wheels
- Health education programs
- Head Start
- WIC (Women's Infants and Children)
- Medical centers/hospitals
- Clinical and food services
- Diabetes centers
- Nursing homes
- Public schools.

Parents who have stayed at home for a couple of years with their children often feel their skills are rusty. Before entering the work force, they may allow some time to do some structured volunteering. It could be as a fund-raiser or a kitchen supervisor at the YMCA. Seek out a not-for-profit organization and offer your professional skills. Offer the skills you feel you need help documenting. One woman wanted to improve her management skills so she would be considered for a new position being planned in her company. She decided to volunteer at a local shelter, managing people, supplies, and money. She used community service as a way of building her skills and proving her abilities to her employer.

In a recent meeting of industry recruiters, several said they look specifically for candidates with community service in their background. They believe individuals who volunteer will be willing to stay a little longer to get the project done; it signals an individual who is interested in giving back to, and not just taking from, the community—even the corporate community. Additionally, community service is another way to create positive public relations. Sometimes people are hired because of their volunteer connections and earned respect in the local or regional community. Other employers will require employees to do some community service such as Big Brother, Big Sister, little league coach, city council members, or serve as the Cancer Society or Heart Association chairperson.

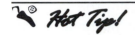 *Hot Tip!*

Many employers will hire a student with lower grades and good volunteer experience over a straight-A student with no volunteerism.

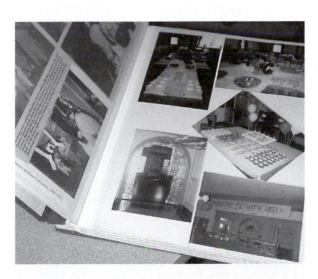

Include pictures of your involvement in community service.

Citizenship, ethics, and the ability to balance your life is becoming more important. Volunteerism shows that you have a strategy for coping with on-the-job stress. Interviewers are looking for ways of seeing balance in your life. Community service is one way to demonstrate this.

- It is appropriate to show work developed while serving with or on community organizations or associations. Examples might include photos of events you assisted with, copies of programs you helped develop or deliver, or samples of the brochures, bylaws, or organizational pieces you developed. Remember, the organizations you associate with are a reflection on you—choose causes you are proud to be associated with over time.

- As your career progresses, you need to keep your samples up to date. Select your most significant contributions as well as those most current from the last 18 months.

Don't underestimate this section of your portfolio. Here is your opportunity. The person reading your portfolio now has the chance to ask questions about you, your values and beliefs. Be sure you associate with causes you can support. It's important to understand the mission statement of the organization even if it's not printed on the brochure. Be prepared to answer questions about your service and about the association or organization.

Dietetic Internship Plan

Include the job description or details that show what you have done in your internship, Depending on your work experiences and education, you may want to create a separate tab in your portfolio for your internship experience. Having all the related materials in the same area of your portfolio can be a great way to support a discussion of your internship during an interview.

Academic Plan of Study

You may be asking why you need to include an academic plan of study. The answer is really quite logical—you want to promote all the specialized education and/or training you have received. It also helps a current or potential employer distinguish between your background and that of other people in the same position. Your plan of study defines the courses you took to complete your degree. Remember that each school, college, or university has a distinct curriculum—you want your program to be known.

DIETETICS OPTION CURRICULUM
Murray State University
P.O. Box 9, Murray, Ky. 42071

1999-2000

University Studies Requirements 47 hours

Communication and Basic Skills 9 hours
___ ENG 101 (3) Composition
___ ENG 102 (3) Composition and Research
___COM 161 (3) Intro Public Speaking
or
___COM 181 (3) Intro Interpersonal Comm

Science and Mathematics: 11 hours
___ BIO 101 (4) Biological Concepts
___CHE 105 (4) Intro Chemistry I or
___CHE 121 (4) General College Chemistry
___MAT 117 (4) Mathematical Concepts (or higher math)

Humanities and Fine Arts 9 hours
___HUM 211 (3) The Western Humanities Tradition
___HUM 212 (3) The Humanities in the Western World
___ ___ ___ (3) Humanities or Fine Arts Elective

Social Sciences 9 hours
___CIV 101 (3) World Civilization and Cultures I
___CIV 102 (3) World Civilization and Cultures II
___PSY 180 (3) General Psychology

University Studies Electives 9 hours
___SOC 133 (3) Intro to Sociology
___CSC 199 (3) Intro to Information Technology
___ (3) Elective

Limited Electives 6 hours (choose from this list or other electives as approved by advisor)
___EXS 250 (3) Fundamentals of Exercise Physiology
___EXS 375 (3) Biokenetics
___EXS 450 (4) Advanced Exercise Physiology
___FCS 111 (3) Family and Its Environment
___FCS 210 (3) Child Development I
___FCS 211 (3) Child Development II
___NTN 597 (1-3) Trends & Issues
___GTY 264 (3) Psychology of Aging
___GTY 305 (3) Services to Older Americans
___GTY 341 (3) Social Gerontology
___BIO 120 (1) Scientific Etymology
___BIO 220 (1) Clinical Terminology
___JMC 168 (3) Contemporary Mass Media
___JMC 194 (3) Newswriting
___NUR 447 (3) Stress Management

Core Requirements 42-44 hours
___NTN 099 (1) Freshman Orientation
___NTN 230 (3) Nutrition
___NTN 231 (4) Princ. of Food Science and Prep
___NTN 233 (3) Nutrition Throughout the Life Cycle
___NTN 235 (2) Quantity Food Production Practicum
___NTN 312 (3) Community Nutrition & Health
___NTN 332 (3) Meal Management Laboratory
___NTN 372 (3) Quantity Food Production. & Purchasing
___NTN 373 (3) Manage. Food Service Personnel & Facilities
___NTN 399 (1) Seminar in Dietetics
___NTN 432 (3) Experimental Foods
___FCS 461 (3) Methods of Teaching
___BPA 140 (3) Foundations of Business
___CHE 210 (3) Brief Organic Chemistry
___MGT 350 (3) Fundamentals of Management
___PSY 300 (3) Principles and Methods of Statistical Analysis
or
___MAT 135 (4) Intro. To Probability & Statistics
or
___CIS 243 (2) Business Statistics I
and
___CIS 343 (2) Business Statistics II

Dietetics Option Requirements 33-34 hours
___BIO 228 (4) Human Anatomy or
___EXS 250 (3) Fundamentals of Exercise Physiology
___BIO 229 (4) Human Physiology
___BIO 300 (4) Intro. Microbiology
___SOC 303 (3) Introduction to Research Methods
___SWK 311(3) Social Work Practice Skills or
___REC 515 (3) Leisure in Therapeutic Recreation Services
___CHE 330 (3) Basic Biochemistry
___NTN 434 (1) Clinical Dietetics Practicum
___NTN 440 (3) Clinical Dietetics
___NTN 532 (3) Advanced Nutrition
___NTN 535 (3) Medical Nutrition Therapy & Diseases
___NTN 536 (3) Methods in Medical Nutrition Therapy

Total Curriculum Requirements 128-132 hours

An Academic Plan of Study helps employers
identify the courses required for your education.

Look to course catalogs for copies of your plan of study. You can also use the description/presentation in the school bulletin or catalog. You need to show all your courses in your major and related area. Be sure to include the pages with the program, department, and degree description, as well as the title page and the date. It may be appropriate to include the course descriptions from key classes. You may need to scan the information. Be sure to cite the date of the program and version of the catalog. You will find all of this especially helpful if you ever go back to school for an advanced degree.

If you are just out of school some employers may ask for a copy of your transcripts. **Transcripts** list the courses you have taken along with your grades. If your grades are not that great, don't volunteer the transcript. You should, however, indicate that it is available upon request. Before you leave your school, get 10 copies of your transcript.

In an interview, the academic plan of study section is usually only referred to if needed and may even be overlooked when the person considering you is reviewing your portfolio. You should have it in your portfolio, just in case.

Faculty and Employer Biographies

Faculty and employer bios are used to give you credibility. The person who signed your skill set sheets or letters of recommendation is giving his or her word that you have certain abilities. The faculty/employer bio sheet gives the interviewer background on who these people are and how they know you.

A faculty/employer bio sheet should include the following information:

- Name and job title
- Organization
- Contact information including address, phone/fax/e-mail
- Areas of specialty
- Date.

The arrangement of bios should be chronological. It is not necessary to repeat a bio for someone unless he or she has been promoted during the signature periods in a skill set.

The employer and faculty bio sheet can be placed under its own tabbed section in the portfolio, following your skill areas. Or you may group it with other reference type materials under an "Additional Materials" tab.

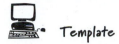 Template

A faculty and employer bio sheet can be found on the enclosed CD. **(Faculty_Employer bios.doc)**

References

You will need three to five references that an employer can check. You should include character, academic, and employment references:

- **Character—** Someone you've worked with in the community, such as church, synagogue or mosque, not-for-profit organizations, clubs, and/or associations can provide good character references.
- **Academic—** Professors, teachers, counselors, coaches, and people who know your academic abilities can provide academic references.
- **Employment—** Supervisors, managers, human resource people at your current and previous positions can provide employment references.

It is never appropriate to use a peer, a subordinate, or a family member as a reference.

Include the person's name, full title, work address, work phone, fax, e-mail, and, if given permission, the person's home phone. Arrange all references on one page, and signal at the bottom of the reference the skills, competencies, or achievements the person can address. If you have more than three references, put them into two columns on the page.

You should be certain each of your references has a copy of your résumé and copies of work samples referred to them. As long as you keep them as a reference, you should forward them a copy of your résumé each time it is updated. Let them know when they may expect to be contacted.

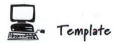 Template

A reference sheet template is included on the enclosed CD. **(References.doc)**

Sample Reference Sheet

June Walsh- References

Ms. Fran Bahmer
General Manager, Heartland Health Services
RR1, Box 50
Bloomington, IL 55555
Office: (309) 663-0000
Fax: (309) 663-0001
(Internship Preceptor)

Dr. George Wilson
Director of Dietetics, Nutrition, and Sports Medicine
211 Park Place
Providence, RI 55555
Office: (123) 456-7890
Fax: (123) 456-9870
E-mail: gwilson@provider.com
Home: (123) 456-4321 (hours: 6 p.m. to 9 p.m.)
(Academic Reference, Club Adviser)

Monsignor Robert McCaffrey
Providence Catholic Diocese
8800 Cathedral Square
Providence, RI 55555
Office: (123) 452-0987
Fax: (123) 452- 9876
(Personal Reference, Community Service)

February, 2004

A sample reference list

Proving Your Worth

Your work samples and support materials make up the largest portion of your portfolio. Take the time to save certificates, samples, and projects as you acquire them. Get into the habit of looking at your work and looking for samples. Take advantage of the moment and take photos of events and projects. Print just one more copy of that report and throw it into your portfolio file. If you don't have many work samples, request letters of recommendation or use skill sets to prove your worth. Once you have these elements together for your portfolio, you're almost ready to begin assembly.

 Taking Action!

Things to do:

- Decide which skill areas you want to promote about yourself
- Start to collect work samples that support your skills
- Track items needed for any professional certifications you may be working on and store them with your other work samples
- Create your own skill sets if needed
- Find your certificates, awards, degrees, and diplomas and make color copies or scan and print them on a color printer.

In your current job:

- Look for work samples you can use in your portfolio
- Ask for letters of recommendation and references as appropriate
- Make a list of your work in progress
- Keep track of any certificates and awards received on the job
- Open the **Faculty_Employer bios.doc** file from the CD and begin to fill out the information about people who are mentioned in your portfolio.

In your school work:

- Look at the projects and assignments that you have completed over your school career. Find samples that show your skills in your key areas.
- Ask for letters of recommendation from teachers.
- Secure any academic references you need for your reference listing.
- Keep track of any certificates and awards received at school.
- Make a copy of your academic plan of study.
- Open the **Faculty_Employer bios.doc** file from the CD and begin to fill out the information about faculty members who are mentioned in your portfolio.

In your volunteer efforts:

- Look at your volunteer experiences and see if you've gained skills you want to promote in your portfolio. Look for work samples you can use: programs, flyers, certificates, photos of yourself in action, etc.
- Ask for a certificate of participation or a letter of recommendation from your volunteer organizations.

In your professional memberships:

- Find your professional membership cards
- Look for work samples from your membership activities
- Ask for letters of recommendation or documentation of your involvement in your professional memberships.

CHAPTER 5

THE ASSEMBLY

Assembling the Portfolio

OK, you have all your stuff in piles and files—now what? Remember, the first chapter of this book gave you the big picture view on the portfolio. Chapters 2 to 4 gave you the gory details of each section in the portfolio (perhaps even more than you really wanted to know). This chapter will take you from the pieces to the whole finished product. You won't be ready to assemble until you first gather, sort, secure, and update your materials. We'll also take a look at special tips for assembling an on-the-job portfolio for use in job reviews or promotion interviews.

Here are the five major steps to assembling your portfolio:

Step 1. Gather your supplies and documents.

Step 2. Sort and organize your work samples.

Step 3. Put them all together in your portfolio.

Step 4. Develop support materials.

Step 5. Check it out— proof it, test it.

Step 1 . . . Things to Gather

If you haven't already done so, read chapters 1 to 4 of this book. Know what your goals and objectives are and how you plan to use your portfolio. Next, bring to one central location all your collected materials—consciously collect:

- Portfolio supplies— (see Chapter 1, "What Supplies Do I Need to Get Started?" or Chapter 9, "Resource Guide")
- Your résumé
- Your brief bio

- Your work philosophy
- Your professional goals
- Your box of work samples... (Are there any old papers or projects that you can find or copy?)
- Certifications
- Degrees or diplomas
- Thank-you letters and letters of recommendation
- Skill sets with signatures
- Faculty/employer bios
- Dietetic Internship plan
- Academic plans of study
- Professional membership cards and service samples
- Certification checklists
- Community service and volunteerism samples
- List of references
- And don't forget—a good friend.

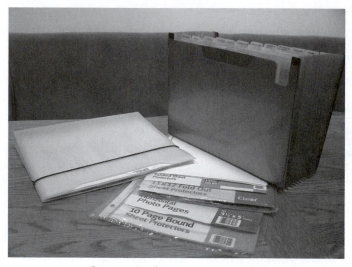

Step 1. Gather your materials.

Assemble Your Portfolio BEFORE You Need It!

With all the work involved in creating a portfolio, it's easy to put it off until another day. If you decide not to choose this option of working in advance on the portfolio, please refer to the Emergency "I Need the Portfolio Now" instructions in chapter 9, "Resource Guide." We promise you'll need them. Even the authors of this book have had to choose between sleep and finishing a portfolio. Be prepared to clean off a big section of the floor or table for the assembly.

Step 2 . . . Sorting and Organizing Work Samples

Set up Your Tabbed Areas

Use the job description, classified ad, and any other knowledge you have of the company or the position to prioritize the skills you will emphasize in your portfolio. Begin by selecting three to five main skill areas you want to emphasize and create a tab for each. Select categories which you can support with work samples. Most dietitians create tabs such as Management, Finance, Clinical, Food Service, Community, Research, or Communication. If you have a certification in a specialty area, you'll probably want to highlight it under its own tab. Now is the time to decide what other tabbed areas beyond work samples you want to use.

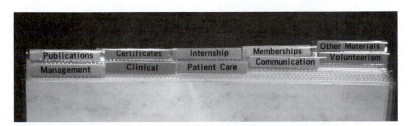

Step 2. Select tabs that represent you.

Remember, this is your portfolio. You need to select the tabbed areas that best represent you. If you don't have any community service experiences, don't create a tab for it and then leave it blank. Don't struggle to find some activity or event to include just so you can write up two lines on a page. If you don't have it, don't include it! Play to your strengths. If you have only one sample for an area, consider grouping it with another sample from a different area and make a tab to reflect this. If you've been on the job for 10 years, you don't need to include a tab for

Academic Plan of Study. You may just want to set up one tab for Additional Materials and place your references list and Faculty and Employer Bio sheet in that section. If you can only come up with two really good tabbed areas, don't struggle to find a third and then include marginal samples. You are designing this portfolio to show off your strengths. Choose your tabbed areas to reflect this.

You also need to create tabs for the other pieces of your portfolio; this may include separate tabs for:

- Work Philosophy and Goals
- Résumé
- Community Service or Volunteerism
- Certificates and Awards
- Professional Memberships
- Academic Plan of Study
- Publications
- Employer and Faculty Bios
- References.

Select Samples

How do you decide which samples to use? Consider first the needs of the employer and look at the job ad to see what samples would be most effective. When sorting work and service samples, ask yourself:

- Which skills is the organization looking for in this position?
- What is your best work?
- Which samples show the most skills and competencies?
- Which work samples are the most interesting to you?
- Which samples are more than just text? Do any include pictures?
- Can you talk about your sample?

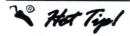 Hot Tip!

Remember to select your best samples!

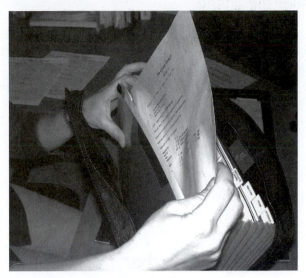

Step 2. Select your best samples.

Consider using some of the following items as demonstrations of your skills and competency:

- Class projects
- Projects or reports demonstrating organization and professionalism
- Writing samples
- Menus created with nutrition software
- Team efforts
- Certificates from workshops
- Performance appraisals (include internships/co-ops)
- Menus created
- Interviews
- Certifications
- Handouts
- Presentations
- Letters itemizing what you have accomplished
- Patient education materials created
- Articles written for magazines and newsletters
- Newspaper articles
- More samples
- Awards and certificates received
- Photos of your volunteer activities.

Remember the Friend

Having a friend there to help you during assembly can be extremely important. Your friend is there to ask the right questions and to look at your portfolio from a different angle. Your friend's job is to ask you the really hard questions that push you to be your best. Your friend is also here to role play possible answers you may give the interviewer. Don't take things personally; give that friend honest answers even if they are not your best answers. You'll improve with practice.

Once you have organized your work samples, you are then ready to develop the support materials that give your portfolio flow.

Step 3 . . . Putting It Together

Now that you have everything gathered, go ahead and put everything you've prepared into page protectors and into the three-ring notebook. Organize your information into appropriate tabbed areas. Remember, we've included several documents on the accompanying diskette that can give you a starting point for creating your documents. Refer to chapter 9, "Resource Guide," for a complete listing of all templates.

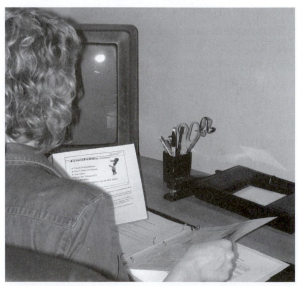

Step 3. Put all your documents in the portfolio.

- Begin with your work philosophy and career goals.
- Put your brief biography in another page protector behind the work philosophy/goals page followed by your résumé.
- Insert skill sets if used.
- Insert letters of recommendation where appropriate.
- Order your work samples and put them into page protectors. You may want to use connected page protectors to keep samples together. Order the work samples with your best examples first.
- Insert copies of certifications, diplomas, and degrees.
- Insert community service samples.
- Insert professional membership certificates and service samples.
- Insert academic plan of study, internship plan, and faculty/employer bios.
- Insert references.

Step 4 . . . Developing Support Materials

Now that you have the key elements inserted into the portfolio, it's time to create a few support materials.

Statement of Originality and Confidentiality

This one-page sheet should be placed at the beginning of your portfolio. It states that the portfolio is your work and indicates if certain portions of the portfolio should not be copied.

Statement of Originality and Confidentiality

This portfolio is the work of Jack Clark, MS, RD. Please do not copy without permission. Some of the exhibits, work samples, and/or service samples are the proprietary property of the organization whose name appears on the document. Each has granted permission for this product to be used as a demonstration of my work.

Sample Statement of Originality and Confidentiality

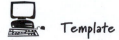 Template

Use the document on the accompanying diskette to create your own page. **(stmt of originality.doc)**

Work Sample Overview Cards

An overview card is a small card (the size of a business card) that contains a brief description of the work sample. Use sheets of blank business cards to print descriptive information about each sample you have within your portfolio. If you have electronic copies of a work sample, you may want to edit the file and insert a text box directly into the work sample to act as your overview card. This way, your overview card remains with the sample at all times.

You may encounter a situation where an electronic work sample does not fill an entire page. In these cases, it is appropriate to add headers to the page (in addition to the overview card) briefly describing what the work sample represents. Whether you choose to print separate overview cards using business cards or insert electronic overview cards, each overview card should include certain details about the work sample:

- Title
- Purpose
- Date developed
- Names of team members who developed it
- Demonstrated skills in keyword format—use words that are emphasized on your résumé and heading.

Nutrition Therapy Brochure

Developed brochure for anyone
making an appointment with the center
June 2004

Skills - Patient communication, organization,
customer focus, creativity

Overview card for a work sample

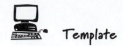 Template

Use the template on the enclosed disk to create your own work sample overview cards. **(Work Sample Overview Cards.doc)**

Allow for Your Style

You are creating a document that represents you and your career to the world. Be sure it feels like you and is a tool you feel comfortable using. Some people make title pages for each section of their portfolios. You can use clip art, photos, and graphics to give the portfolio your own style. Just be sure the end result looks professional. No dancing broccoli or singing carrots please!

General Rules to Follow

- Put all papers into the page protectors using both the front and back
- Use colored paper to draw attention to special work or service samples
- Use the same type of paper on your résumé and references (prepare two extra sets of these documents to hand out during the interview)
- Proofread everything at least three times
- NEVER USE YOUR ORIGINALS
- Refer to Chapter 8, "A Matter of Style," for details on making your portfolio look its best.

Step 5 . . . Check It Out

We hope this was not an emergency assembly of your portfolio and that you have at least 12 hours to proof and let the portfolio cool. Here are a few items you should check and recheck:

- Read for typos, spelling, grammar, and format. If you are not good at this, have a friend do it.
- Talk through the sections of your portfolio with a friend, thinking about which parts you will elaborate on in an interview.

- When in doubt, take it out . . . if you are not sure or are not pleased with an item—leave it out.
- If you have assembled this portfolio for a particular interview, make sure you have selected work samples that meet the needs of the organization.

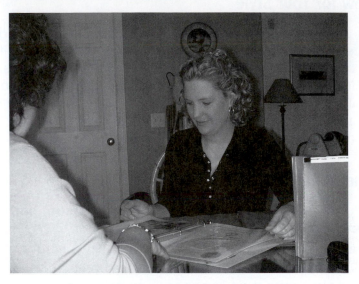

Step 5. Review your portfolio with a friend.

Assembling an On-the-Job Portfolio

When you have a job, your portfolio can help you keep it and get a pay increase or promotion. The overall organization of the portfolio is the same, except that work samples are organized in chronological order and your professional goals may be organized by your previous year's professional goals and objectives (or the time since your last appraisal).

- **Check your calendar—** Get in the habit of writing down the start dates, benchmarks, and completion dates of projects. Write down on your calendar any letters of acknowledgment or awards received. Months from now you will have a road map ready to read and secure your documentation for the portfolio.
- **Once a month make two lists of what you have accomplished, planned and unplanned—** If you can't do it

once a month, then take 30 minutes once every 90 days and think about your career. Make the appointment with yourself right now; map out the appointments and keep them.

- **Set up a file box or file drawer—** At the end of each project, make a second copy of it and put it in your file. At the very least, save it on a disk. Remember that setting aside a copy of your work needs to become reflex; it will save you a lot of chasing when you put together your actual portfolio.

- **Review the job description for your position—** As far in advance of the review as possible, reread your job description. Use the job description to guide your search for work samples. You may even want to consider seeking out certifications that will document and help you recover from any deficits. If you don't have a specific job description for your position (and many people don't), write your own. Give a copy of your job description to your supervisor and seek his or her input. It is helpful and strategic to establish the criteria of your position before your review.

- **Review the performance appraisal standards before the actual review—** It seems simple, but be sure you understand the rules of the game at the beginning of the performance period. This may or may not be possible. Some organizations have very general standards or criteria. Now that you know the specifics, keep them in the back of your mind as you make decisions on your work samples and career activities.

- **Concentrate on your skill sets, your work samples, and professional activities—** The other parts of the portfolio, such as your work philosophy, goals, résumé, awards, and certificates, should appear in your portfolio but not be emphasized. These sections serve as background and quite often serve as subtle support to refresh the reviewer's knowledge of you.

- **Put it all together—** Put together this year's work in chronological order or into the major areas set up in your job description. Then be sure to explain to the person reviewing you that you have put together a self-review. Set your supervisor up to use your career portfolio. Don't just walk in the door with your portfolio; it could be perceived as a threat. Always explain your portfolio before you use it.

Congratulations—You Have a Career Portfolio!

Whew!! Assembly is a lot of work. If you've gotten to this point and have a finished portfolio in hand, congratulate yourself. You've taken a huge step toward understanding yourself, and you're ready to take your portfolio to the marketplace. You have taken time to examine your beliefs and goals and had the opportunity to evaluate your work, your skills, your strengths and weaknesses. You've searched through and found the best examples of your work and you now have a tool for tracking your career.

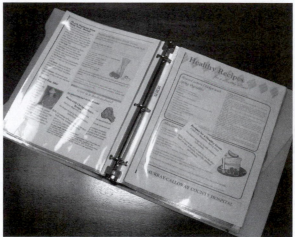

The finished portfolio involves a lot of hard work!

In the next chapter, we'll look at how you can adapt your portfolio into an electronic portfolio. If you want to explore the new frontier of Internet web sites and find ways to create new opportunities, read on. If you can't wait to learn how to actually use your portfolio in an interview or a job review, or to complete your internship application, go on to Chapter 7, "The Portfolio in Action."

Taking Action!

Things to do when assembling your portfolio:

- Schedule a time in your calendar to assemble your portfolio
- Purchase any supplies needed to complete your portfolio
- Take time to sort and organize your work samples into key skill areas
- Make copies of any documents you want to include (Don't include your originals!!)
- Create tabs for each section of your portfolio
- Put all documents into sheet protectors
- Use the template on the CD **(stmt of originality.doc)** to create your Statement of Originality and Confidentiality
- Use the business card template on the CD **(Work Sample Overview Cards.doc)** to create overview cards for each work sample
- Proofread all your materials, checking for spelling and grammar.

If you're assembling a portfolio for a performance appraisal:

- Schedule time every month to review your work to look for work samples for your portfolio
- Keep a copy of your work samples in a folder to use when you assemble your portfolio
- Review your work goals to identify work samples
- Be sure to assemble your portfolio well in advance of your review meeting so your boss has time to review your portfolio ahead of time.

CHAPTER 6

THE ELECTRONIC PORTFOLIO

Technology Levels the Playing Field

What exactly is an electronic career portfolio? It is a personalized, career-oriented web site that you use to get a job or to make your skills known. It can be accessed from the Internet, or you can control access to the portfolio by putting it on a disk or CD-ROM. The electronic career portfolio contains the same information as your "hard copy" portfolio, but it is organized and accessed differently. Consider this . . . the hard copy portfolio is linear, like a newspaper which is read one page after the other. The electronic portfolio is nonlinear, or organized in such a way you can access a page or sample from several different pages. There is no specific order in which you have to view the pages.

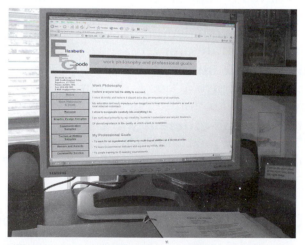

Electronic portfolios can be stored on a web site,
a CD-ROM, Zip, or floppy disk.

Why Would I Want an Electronic Portfolio?

"It takes long enough to develop a hard copy portfolio, why would I want to spend all my time developing a web site to do the same thing?" You're asking the right question. The beauty of the electronic portfolio is its ability to:

- **Cluster ideas that are related—** Consider using the same work sample but showing your link in two or more skill areas. For example, you may have a report you generated which shows your leadership ability, nutritional assessment, knowledge of technology, and training skills. If you have separate pages for leadership, technology, and training, you can reference the same sample from each page. You are able to dial in the user to the exact parts of the work sample with the electronic portfolio.

- **Be quickly scanned and searched—** You can set up buttons (like tabs) to easily access key information.

- **Add more of yourself—** As your voice or a video clip. Short sound bites allow you to "show yourself in action." Keep in mind these files can be big and work fine on a CD but may be too big or take too long for access on a web connection. Make sure to have appropriate permissions from the hospital or company before filming or photographing anyone. Remember there are strict confidentiality laws involving patients and company/corporate property.

- **Follow up your interview with support material—** It is appropriate to leave a "copy" of your career portfolio in electronic form for an interviewer to review at a later time.

- **Provide new and different work samples that supplement your hard copy portfolio—** You can include more work samples in the electronic portfolio that support your paper portfolio.

So . . . Do I Even Need a Paper Career Portfolio?

Oh, yes! The hard copy and the electronic portfolio include the same elements, but people process, view, and explore the information differently. The paper (hard copy) portfolio and the electronic portfolio work differently in the career market.

Hard Copy Portfolios

- Hard copies work better in interviews. They are more flexible and easier to manage in an interview setting. They allow you to interact with the interviewer in a personal way.

- Some people may not have access or be comfortable using a computer.

- It is usually faster to make changes to a hard copy portfolio by switching out work samples to meet the needs of an interview. It takes more time to adjust the contents of an electronic portfolio.

When Does the Electronic Portfolio Become Attractive?

- As follow up after a successful interview—so others who did not get time to spend with you can be SOLD on you

- When they want more time with you after the interview to learn even more about you

- It is something they can view without time restrictions

- It is a perk that you have some technology literacy.

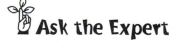 Ask the Expert

When to use an electronic portfolio

Q. Is it appropriate to use an electronic portfolio during an interview?

A. Typically you do not use an electronic portfolio during an interview unless you are interviewing for a position in the tech field. The paper portfolio lends itself best to the needs of an interview. There are three ways a paper portfolio is used in an interview:

1. Offer your portfolio at the beginning of an interview for the interviewer to review.

2. Use your portfolio to answer a question during your interview.

3. Use your portfolio as a summary or review at the end of the interview.

An electronic portfolio is best used during the pre-interview process by noting on your cover letter that you have a portfolio available for preview. It can also be an effective tool after an interview as a summary.

Some things to keep in mind regarding your electronic portfolio include:

- Make it easy to navigate; set it up to automatically start
- Be sure to attach the directions for launching the electronic portfolio
- Common platforms for an electronic portfolio include using PowerPoint slides or HTML (web page) formats.

Electronic Portfolios Work Differently

Electronic portfolios are used differently than printed ones—you can't expect the person to whom you are showing it to run and get his/her laptop. You can, however, use it as the copy you leave with the interviewer to support your printed copy. People process information differently, and tabbed work samples and statements support what you say. With the electronic portfolio and the nonlinear approach, you can never be sure in what order people will view your info—so it becomes more important that it be able to stand alone and is organized into chunks.

Wait! I'm Not a "Techno-Wizard"— How Can I Do This?

If you're feeling a little intimidated right now, thinking you don't have the skills or ability to design a web site or something really technical . . . relax. There are several ways to get this accomplished and it doesn't have to cost a lot. You are either going to design this web site yourself or you're going to get someone to help you. There are actually many easy-to-use programs for designing web sites where you don't have to know any "code" or "HTML" stuff, and some are even free.

Stay focused on your goal. If you have problems "coding" or getting something to work like a graphic or a table or a form, call in your "tech" buddies or friends for help. Don't let the technology manage you. Don't give up. Local universities have plenty of places with lab assistance. If you are in school, check out job boards and find a person who is looking for a way to get more web development experience for their portfolio! You can also hire someone to create a site. Look for students who are studying multimedia or web design.

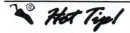

You can easily convert documents in Microsoft Word, PowerPoint, Excel, and Publisher directly into web pages through the software.

Getting It All Together

- **What do you already have on disk?**— Find projects, case studies, educational in-services, reports, presentations, budgets, etc., that you already have in electronic format.

- **Get the rest of your documents into electronic format**— (Take your tote box to a friend with a scanner!) This can take some time, so allow half a day or so for this task.

- **Get yourself an electronic suitcase**— Find a way to store all these files. You can put files on several diskettes, a Zip disk, a writable/rewritable CD-ROM disk, or have someone burn a CD-ROM disk for you with all your samples.

- **Get the software you will use to develop the web page and figure out how to use it**— or get your techno friend to help.

- **Not all work samples belong on your electronic portfolio**— Prioritize and choose your best samples. You may need to customize your electronic portfolio for a potential employer, so scan all of your work samples.

- **Now you're ready to design your site!**

Designing the Electronic Career Portfolio

- Start with a solid, working hard copy career portfolio.
- Consider your style and your "look," including:
    - ◆ Fonts
    - ◆ White space
    - ◆ Graphics and photos.

- Decide how you will structure the items to be used, including Work Samples, Work Philosophy, Goals, Résumé, References, Certificates, etc. Will they go on separate pages, or will some of them be together?

- Use templates and wizards where possible. A template for the electronic career portfolio is included on the CD in a directory called **e_portfolio**.

- Choose the work samples—remember that you can organize them in a nonlinear way.

- Storyboard the electronic portfolio; that is to say, take a large sheet of paper and colored markers or pencils and draw pictures of what you want where and what links or references you want on the contained pages. If you have access to a classroom or boardroom, use the chalk or white board. Take a good look here at how much information you want to give in the "big" picture. How much information do you want to have connected and how do you want the people to navigate or move through your portfolio? Consider using basic web HTML editors.

- Design the site on your computer.

- Test it to make sure it works. Pull in a few friends and have them take a look. Revise the site as needed.

- Write the instructions for executing the files. Attach them to the holder of your disk or the cover letter with your web site.

- Then go for it—electronically produce the portfolio, date, and make copies. If you have to acquire a new skill, consider how it will support you in your career. In today's world most people are used to navigating a web site and understand how they work.

- Once you've developed a web site on your computer, you need to get it from your computer to the Internet. Keep in mind that when it's on the Internet, everyone can access it unless you know how to password protect it.

- You need to find a host for your web site. There are a lot of free or inexpensive ways. First, check with your Internet service provider (ISP) to see if you can put up a free personal web site—many ISPs include a "personal" site as part of your monthly fee. You can also get space on other sites. Many colleges and universities offer free web space for every student.

Upload Your Files

- Once you've got a place to put your site, you need to "upload" your files from the computer to the web. This process is called FTPing, or publishing your files. Most ISPs will provide clear directions and help for people new to the process.

- You will be given a user name and password that will allow you to upload the files to a specific location on the web site. To update the site you make changes to the pages on your computer and then upload the files to the web. If you know how to copy and paste files between directories on a computer, you can update your site. If you need assistance, find a friend to help, or pay someone to help you. The finished site must look professional.

Maintaining Your Site

- Put up current work samples as you create them.
- Don't forget to take it down. When you get the job or achieve the goal it may be time to take down your site. You don't want to generate "business" if you're unable to accept it.

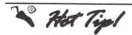 Hot Tip!

Don't forget to include your web address in your hard copy portfolio!

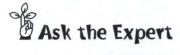

Ask the Expert

Publicizing your site

Q. Should I include the web address in my résumé?

A. It depends on how well dialed in you are to this particular employer. It's very tempting on the electronic portfolio to put more there than you need. You still need to strategically design the web site to meet the needs of the employer.

Making the Most of Your Electronic Portfolio

In all cases, electronic or paper, the career portfolio is a tool for demonstrating who you are and what knowledge and skills you have—use the portfolio to help people learn about you and your attitude. The mental process of developing a career portfolio is the same for a paper hard copy and an electronic portfolio. The real benefit of the electronic portfolio is the ability to give people more time to access your portfolio. For examples of electronic portfolios visit our web site: **http://learnovation.com**

The following pages show pages from a student electronic portfolio. This site was created in Macromedia's Dreamweaver, but you can easily create web pages in Microsoft Publisher, Microsoft Word, and Microsoft FrontPage. You can see this student web site online at **http://learnovation.com/dieteticportfolio/default.htm**

Note: Portions of this electronic portfolio sample have been modified or edited for learning purposes.

 Template

The enclosed disk contains a directory called **e_portfolio**. It contains nine HTML pages you can use to create and customize your own career portfolio. The following pages are included: home/opening page, work philosophy and goals, résumé, four blank skill area pages that can be customized to your specific skill areas, awards, and community service. The style of the pages is similar to the examples on the next few pages. Feel free to change the layout, colors, and information included to create your own unique portfolio.

Home Page

The home page of your web site serves as a starting point for the electronic portfolio. It introduces who you are and serves to orient the viewer to your web site. Navigation buttons help the viewer easily go between the pages in the web site. Underlined text are links to additional pages. The user can click on the text to go to a related page. It is a good idea to put your contact information on the home page, or on a separate contact page.

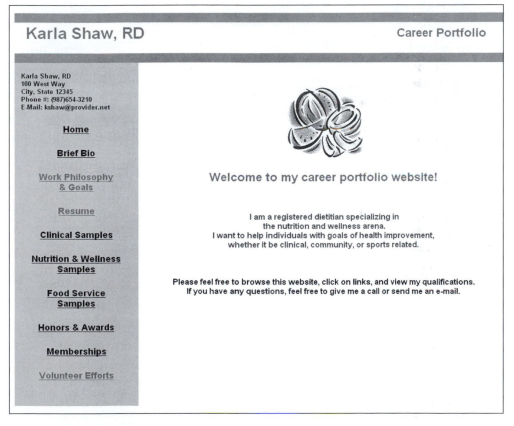

Home page

Work Philosophy and Goals

The following screen shows Karla's work philosophy and goals. This should be one of the first things a person sees when viewing your electronic portfolio. You may choose to list the work philosophy and goals on your home page. You might also decide to add some simple clip art or a photo to make a page more interesting. Be sure any clip art you use is tasteful and related to the items on the page.

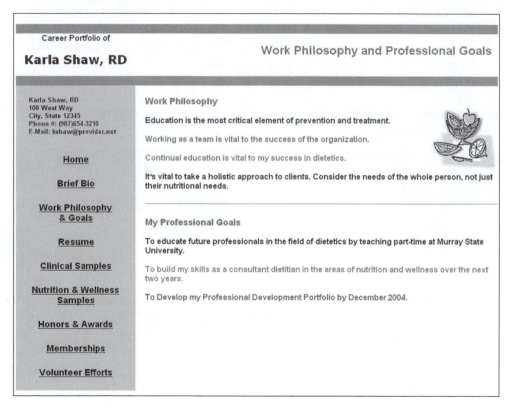

Work philosophy and goals page

Brief Biography

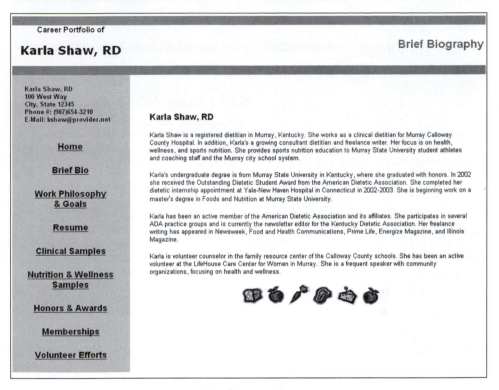

Brief Biography

Career Portfolio of

Karla Shaw, RD

Karla Shaw, RD
100 West Way
City, State 12345
Phone #: (987)654-3210
E-Mail: kshaw@provider.net

Home

Brief Bio

Work Philosophy
& Goals

Resume

Clinical Samples

Nutrition & Wellness
Samples

Honors & Awards

Memberships

Volunteer Efforts

Karla Shaw, RD

Karla Shaw is a registered dietitian in Murray, Kentucky. She works as a clinical dietitian for Murray Calloway County Hospital. In addition, Karla's a growing consultant dietitian and freelance writer. Her focus is on health, wellness, and sports nutrition. She provides sports nutrition education to Murray State University student athletes and coaching staff and the Murray city school system.

Karla's undergraduate degree is from Murray State University in Kentucky, where she graduated with honors. In 2002 she received the Outstanding Dietetic Student Award from the American Dietetic Association. She completed her dietetic internship appointment at Yale-New Haven Hospital in Connecticut in 2002-2003. She is beginning work on a master's degree in Foods and Nutrition at Murray State University.

Karla has been an active member of the American Dietetic Association and its affiliates. She participates in several ADA practice groups and is currently the newsletter editor for the Kentucky Dietetic Association. Her freelance writing has appeared in Newsweek, Food and Health Communications, Prime Life, Energize Magazine, and Illinois Magazine.

Karla is volunteer counselor in the family resource center of the Calloway County schools. She has been an active volunteer at the LifeHouse Care Center for Women in Murray. She is a frequent speaker with community organizations, focusing on health and wellness.

Brief biography page

The brief bio is a short overview of yourself in narrative format. Some people place their bio on their home page as an introduction to themselves. Others make it a separate page. Include a direct link to your résumé from your brief bio. You may also want to hyper link different key terms in your bio if you could link them directly to samples or sections in your portfolio.

Résumé

The résumé on the following two pages looks very similar to Karla's hard copy résumé. She has added colored headings and included links to work samples in other areas of the electronic portfolio. If you click on the "community outreach" link under her current position, you will go to the Community Service page.

Karla Shaw, RD

Resume

Karla Shaw, RD
100 West Way
City, State 12345
Phone #: (987)654-3210
E-Mail: kshaw@provider.net

 Print a copy
(PDF)

Home

Brief Bio

Work Philosophy & Goals

Resume

Clinical Samples

Nutrition & Wellness Samples

Honors & Awards

Memberships

Volunteer Efforts

Karla Shaw, RD

100 West Way• city, state, zip
Phone: (987) 654-3210 • Fax: (123) 456-7891 • E-Mail: kshaw@provider.net

Skills and Qualities

- **Registered dietitian**
- **Self-motivated, creative, problem solver with a "can-do" attitude**
- **Multilingual:** Able to read, write, and speak Spanish fluently
- **Skilled in the following:**
  o ServeSafe - Food Safety Certification - 2004
  o Automated External Defibrillation Training, 2003, 2004
  o C.P.R. Certified, 1998-2003
- **Computer Software:** Microsoft Office, Front Page, Filemaker Pro, Nutrikids, Calendar Maker, Nutritionist Five, Nutriquest
- **Media:** Writing, brochure creation

Education

Dietetic Internship - Yale-New Haven Hospital, New Haven, CT
Post graduate 12 month supervised practice program - September 30, 2002 to September 8, 2003

- Gained experience caring for patients within general medical, cardiology, geriatric, oncology,
  pediatric, psychiatric, renal, maternal, and outpatient settings under the guidance of experienced registered dietitians.

Bachelor of Science - Murray State University Murray, KY
Major: Nutrition and Food Science - Degree: June 2002

- Emphasis in clinical nutrition, wellness, and sports nutrition

Employment

Clinical Dietitian
Murray Calloway County Hospital Murray, KY
November 2003 - Present

- Responsible for nutrition education of patient, patient's families, staff, and students.
- Made recommendations to maintain/improve patient's nutritional status.
- Planned menus to conform to physician's diet order.
- Provided nutrition education to the community as requested.
- Assisted with the education / training of food service employees to ensure high standards in nutrition care.
- Provided sports nutrition education to Murray State University student-athletes and coaching staff, Calloway County School
  system, Murray City School system, and community, as requested.
- Served on following teams / committees as assigned: Quest for Quality team, Courtesy Commando team, JCAHO Key
  Function Care of the Patient committee, Diabetes Recognition team.
- Teach Diabetes Self-Management Classes.

Student Health Liason
Murray State University, Murray Health Center.
September 2001 - September 2002

- Responsible for assisting students with health and wellness inquiries.
- Performed diet analysis on student three day food records.
- Assisted with various presentations, health fairs, promotions regarding nutrition and health related issues.
- Developed handouts, posters and bulletins for promoting health and wellness.
- Conducted presentations in student dormitories to promote low-fat living.

Résumé page

Wellness Counselor
Grant County W.I.C. Office, Murray, KYJanuary 2000 - September 2002, Part Time

- Assisted with various one-on-one counseling sessions with dietitians and nutrition assistants by observing and translating in Spanish.
- Attended various nutrition education classes for WIC participants.
- Became familiar with ISIS database used for tracking WIC participants.
- Developed an Access database and assisted with researching participants for a breastfeeding study.
- Assisted with developing a class outline and reading materials for raising participant awareness about local Farmer's Markets.

Dietetic Aide
St. Elizabeth Hospital, Lexington, KY
June 1996– August 1998

- Analyzed and revised patient menus according to patient needs
- Calculated daily nutrient requirements for patients
- Forecasted inventory needs and placed orders for Food and Nutrition Department

Honors & Awards

- Outstanding Dietetic Student Award, American Dietetic Association - June 2002
- National College Honor Scholarship Society Alpha Chi Member - 2001 - 2002
- National Honor Society Member - 2001-2002
- Scholarship Award - American Dietetic Association - June 1999

Memberships

- American Dietetic Association member (1999 - present)
- Kentucky Dietetic Association member (2000 - present)
  - Student Liason, 2001-2002
  - Newsletter Editor, 2004-2005
- American Culinary Federation (2002 - present)
- American Dietetic Association Practice Group membership:
  - Dietitians in Nutrition Support, 2003
  - Sports, Cardiovascular, and Wellness Nutritionists, 2003 - present
  - Nutrition Entrepreneurs Dietetic Practice Group (2003 - present)

Publications

- "Cooking Solo". AHF Magazine, April/May 2004
- Healthy Recipes for Energize Magazine - Spring 2003 and Spring 2004
- "National Diet-Out Day". Communicating Food for Health, Food and Health Communications, Inc., May 2003.
- "Peanut Power" - Special Advertising Section of Newsweek - April 2003
- Healthy Recipes for Prime Life Magazine - Spring 2003 and Spring 2004
- "Shopping for Weight Loss" Slide Show. Communicating Food for Health, Food and Health Communications, Inc., Jan. 2003.
- "New Year's Res-oat-lutions". Communicating Food for Health, Food and Health Communications, Inc., Jan 2003.
- "Make It A Healthy Holiday". Illinois Magazine, Schuster Media Group, Inc., Nov 2002; 37-39.

Community Service

- Couselor in the Family Resource Center - Calloway County Schools - 2003-present
- Presentation on allergy awareness to IL HeadStart Organization - April 2004
- Nutrition Presentation to State Legislators - April 2004
- Medical Nutrition Therapy for the Treatment of Overweight and Obesity – presentation for Northwestern Memorial Hospital Sleep Clinic - February 2004
- Guest speaker "Eating Disorders: Awareness and Prevention" at local schools, fall 2003
- American Cancer Society Relay for Life participant, 1997-2003
- LifeHouse Care Center for Women, volunteer 1999-2000
  LifeHouse Walk participant, 1999-2001

Résumé page (continued)

The formatting of the online résumé takes up more space and if you print the web page, you may lose some of the information from the printed page. Karla has included a graphic of a printer that is linked to a PDF copy of her résumé. When you click the printer, a new browser window will open and display a printable version of her portfolio in Acrobat Reader. The person viewing the electronic portfolio must have Acrobat Reader installed on their machine in order to view the printable résumé. Acrobat Reader is available for free from Adobe. Most new computers come with Acrobat Reader already installed. In order to make a PDF, you need to have a copy of the complete Adobe Acrobat on your computer.

Key Skill Areas

The next several pages of the electronic portfolio are Karla's key skill areas. These are the skills she is trying to promote to potential employers. She has grouped work samples by area. She has included smaller graphics (sometimes called thumbnails) of her work samples on each page. If the viewer wants to see a larger copy, they can click on the sample, or on the underlined link, and a new window will open with a larger version of the sample. Having documents in a PDF format allows people to print the samples and view them offline. It also keeps the formatting of your documents and allows them to print properly. As with a hard copy portfolio, you should put your most important and best work samples first. You should also organize your key areas, so your strongest area is the first in the site navigation. Additional work samples could include reports, project summaries, slides, and presentations. Remember, the web is visual. People get bored very easily with loads of heavy text. Use graphics and clip art to make your site interesting.

Karla Shaw, RD

Clinical Samples

Karla Shaw, RD
100 West Way
City, State 12345
Phone #: (987)654-3210
E-Mail: kshaw@provider.net

Home

Brief Bio

**Work Philosophy
& Goals**

Resume

Clinical Samples

**Food Service
Samples**

Honors & Awards

Memberships

Volunteer Efforts

I am dedicated to bringing the best service to patients and clients.

(Click on a document to view a PDF of the item)

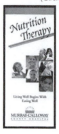

Brochure designed for incoming clients

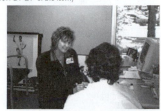

Counseling patients and clients

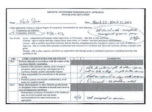

Clinical evaluation forms from my
dietetic internship

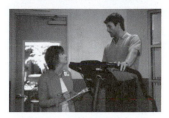

Case study on Medicine rotation

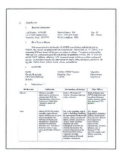

Case study on Onocology rotation

Key skill area - clinical

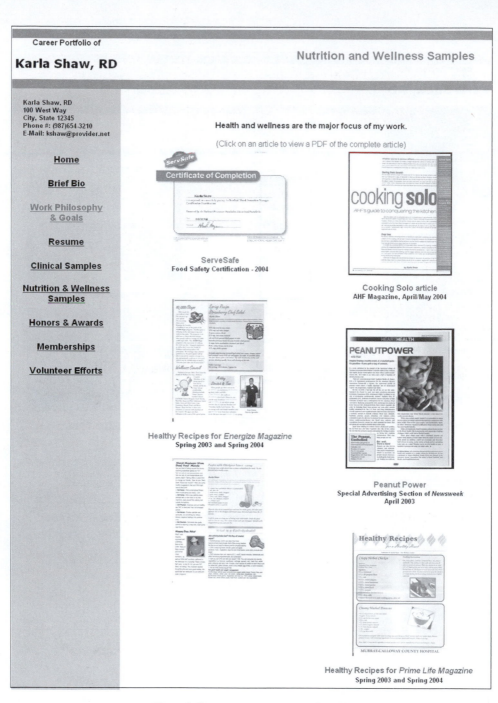

Key skill area - nutrition and wellness

Professional Memberships

Include a page for your involvement in professional organizations. Include membership cards, thank yous, letters of recommendation or participation, or photos of an event or presentation you gave. Include any leadership roles you may have in an organization.

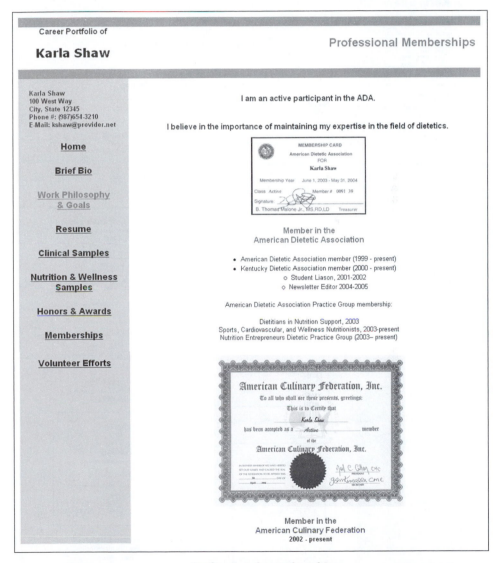

Professional memberships

Honors and Awards

Don't forget to include graphics or photos of honors and awards you've received. Remember, the goal is to show the viewer what sets you apart from others.

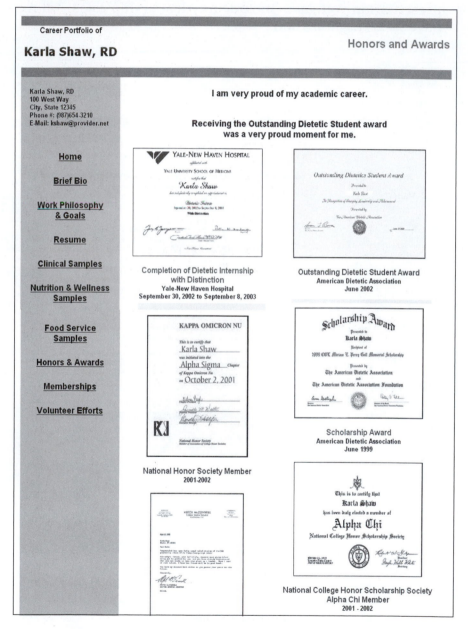

Honors and awards

Community Service/ Volunteerism

Community service is a great place to include certificates and photos of people in action. Don't forget to include graphics and pictures when you can. It makes the electronic portfolio more interesting and draws the viewer into the portfolio.

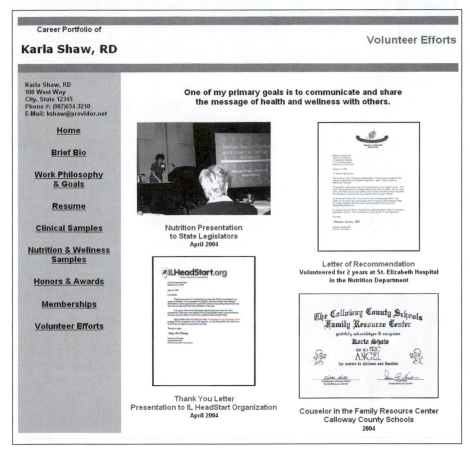

Community service

If you've taken the time to create an electronic portfolio, give yourself a pat on the back—you deserve it! Electronic portfolios give you more flexibility and more opportunities to show your skills and talents, but it takes time and effort to produce an electronic portfolio.

Don't forget that electronic portfolios are often used to give an employer another look at your skills, or to emphasize something you forgot you had. It may be just that extra effort and initiative that gets you into the job you want.

 Taking Action!

Things to do:

- Decide if you want to set up and design your e-portfolio or if you want someone else to do it for you
- Decide how many pages of information to include in the e-portfolio
- Decide on the navigation of the site (How will a person move through the pages?)
- Convert any documents to an electronic format
- Use the blank e-portfolio HTML files on the CD as a starting place for creating your own portfolio
- Place your e-portfolio on a diskette or CD, or upload it to a web server
- Keep your e-portfolio updated and current.

CHAPTER 7

THE PORTFOLIO IN ACTION

Now That I Have It, How Do I Use It?

Now that you have the portfolio, what do you do with it? It looks good, feels nice, and you survived the assembly process. You may be wondering "How do I use this portfolio?" and "How do I let them (the interviewer or boss) know that I have it?" This chapter talks about using your portfolio:

- To set the interviewer up to look at your portfolio
- As an overview of your abilities
- To answer a question
- To get a dietetic internship or practicum
- To demonstrate your abilities in a performance review
- To obtain a promotion.

Interview Techniques

Your portfolio is finished . . . you have assembled work samples and support materials to help you prove to a potential employer that you are the right person for the job. Now, how do you use it? The first thing you need to do is test drive your portfolio before your first interview.

Good marketing is required of you and your work. Promote your portfolio ahead of time by placing a note at the bottom of your résumé: *Professional Portfolio Available upon Request.* You should also refer to the portfolio in your cover letter and on phone interviews when communicating with a company. Your portfolio is one of the prominent tools you take to the interview.

Get Comfortable with Your Portfolio

After assembling the portfolio, you should be intimately acquainted with it. You should know the contents of each tabbed area and be able to explain the significance of each piece of the portfolio. You should be able to tell the interviewer your work philosophy and goals without looking, and you should be able to turn to any work sample and talk about it: what it represents, how it was created, what skills you used during the process, the people involved in developing it, and what you learned from the project. The order of the tabbed areas should be second nature so you aren't flipping through the pages trying to find a particular sample or a certain skill set.

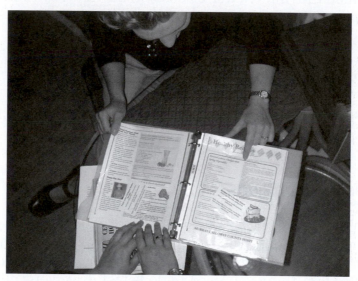

Grab a friend and test drive your portfolio before you need it!

When you can comfortably navigate your portfolio, it's time to try it out on someone else. Grab a friend (preferably the one who helped you assemble your portfolio) and go through a few "mock" interviews. Have your friend ask you common interview questions and practice using the portfolio to provide the answers. You should also practice explaining at the beginning of an interview that you have a portfolio of your work and exactly what that is.

Customize as Needed

Next, you need to get ready for your first interview. You need to research the company and the position and have a good idea of the requirements of the job. You should be able to identify what strengths you bring to the position and what challenges you may have to face in terms of experience or education needs. This is the time to customize your portfolio to the needs of the potential employer.

- If you customized the career objective on your résumé for this company, be sure the copy in your portfolio matches the copy sent to the company.

- You may want to tweak your career goals slightly to take into account any special needs or opportunities presented by the employer.

- Customize your work samples based on the position and the company. If this position requires good training skills, you may want to pull in that training program sample you developed for a management class or a training outline you used when you taught customer service skills. If it is focusing on management skills, you might insert a copy of SWOT analysis or the project timelines you developed in your internship. Choose the work samples that will help you connect with the interviewer. Be prepared to show them why you are the person for the position.

Working the Portfolio in the Interview

During the interview, it's important to let the interviewer know within the first 15 minutes that you have a portfolio available. Watch the interviewer for signals of interest. Use the portfolio to set up the interviewer to ask you the questions you want to answer and that you can answer best. If you are offered the opportunity to overview your portfolio, be conscious of time. In a 30-minute interview. you should be able to overview your portfolio in five to eight minutes, unless there are questions being asked.

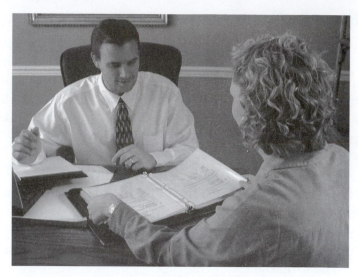

Orient the interviewer to your portfolio.

Actually showing the portfolio may seem physically awkward. You may be sitting opposite the person by the time you are ready to show the portfolio. You may want to get up and stand beside the person to talk briefly through the sections. Make sure your head is not above the interviewer's head. Kneel or bend down to accomplish this. Usually the person viewing it will already be seated. It's difficult to read upside down, so you may want to get up and stand next to the person or people interviewing you. (A gentle reminder—women should pay attention to their necklines when leaning over. Both men and women should be sure their deodorant is working!) If getting up and moving around is not feasible or comfortable for you, you can work the portfolio across a desk. Just be sure the interviewer can clearly see the contents of the portfolio.

- **Begin by overviewing your work philosophy and professional goals—** This shows you have plans and focus— spend a little time here.
- **Point out your résumé and remind the person that he or she already has a copy—** Of course you should have a spare résumé tucked in the inside pocket of the portfolio.
- **For each additional section, describe briefly what the viewer or reader will find—** Let the viewer determine how much detail to go into in each section.

- **Don't use the portfolio to shut off questions from the recruiter**— Give enough overview to pique the person's curiosity so he or she can ask better questions of you. When you're finished showing the portfolio, leave it in front of the person.

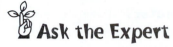

Ask the Expert

Interviewing advice

Q. I am about to graduate from college and am setting up interviews with potential employers. What is your BEST advice for interviewing to help me set myself apart from other applicants?

A. Your career portfolio is a great tool to strengthen an interview. It does a couple of things: first, it helps to guide those interviewers who may not be especially good at conducting interviews, by showing them your work samples and giving insight into you. Second, it helps people, who are not perhaps as outgoing, to anticipate questions as well as to use props to answer. The process of assembling a portfolio gets you to review what you have to offer and to organize it into categories that can increase what you are worth to an employer. When you are asked questions in the interview, you can then show and tell what you know—allowing your work to do some of the speaking for you. Assembling your work samples into key skill areas is the first place to start. Dialing into the culture and goals of the organization also helps one to choose work samples for effectiveness. Community service is also a way to show how well you work with people and contribute to the community.

Emphasis on Course Work

If within the first five minutes of the interview the person has not expressed an interest in the portfolio, be prepared to use it as a means for answering a specific question. It should be easy to answer these questions because you had to answer the same types of questions when you developed your portfolio. Use your classroom projects and course materials to demonstrate your abilities. Here are some questions that lend themselves to be answered by a look at your portfolio:

- **"What are your five-year goals?"** or **"What are your future plans?"** (See the work philosophy and professional goals section.)

- **"How confident are you on the computer?"** (See the work/ service samples with projects that are computer- generated, demonstrating the software and skills they want to see such as spreadsheets, word processing and database project, or any specialty software.)

- **"What do you do for recreation or release?"** (Show them your community service section.)

- **"What was your most challenging case study?"** (Show them a work sample from your class or a case study from an internship rotation.)

- **"Have you ever . . . ?"** (Fill in the blank and show the person a work or service sample.)

- **What certifications do you hold?** (See the certifications, diplomas, and degrees sections.)

- **"How do you work as part of a team?"** (Show them work samples that you generated as a group project and discuss the group dynamics.)

Don't be surprised if the interviewer asks to see the entire portfolio and not just the one section you are showing him or her.

Reactions . . .

You may find the interviewer has never heard about using a portfolio before. Additionally, he or she may not have the time to view it or he or she may be on a tight time schedule and have a list of fixed questions to address. Try to use your portfolio to answer questions. This can often spark the interest of the interviewer. On the other hand, you may find yourself leading the interview through the use of your portfolio. If you are being interviewed by several people in a group setting, you may find the interviewers fight over the opportunity to see your portfolio first. You may be in a situation where you are talking to one person and another person is looking at your portfolio. Using the work sample overview cards in each page can help a person understand the contents of your portfolio without your aid. This may be helpful.

Normally, you will be able to find some way to work the portfolio into the interview or review. However, if you do not spark the interviewer's interest, even after a clear offering and explanation of what the portfolio is, trust your instincts. It may be that going through the process improved your interviewing skills enough that they are intimidated by your organization.

Leaving Your Portfolio

If you have sparked the curiosity of the interviewer with your portfolio, he or she may ask you to leave it with the company overnight so they can review it in more detail. If this is feasible and you have no other interviews in the time frame, it may be a great opportunity to reinforce your abilities to the interviewer. Make sure you clearly arrange a time to pick up the portfolio when he or she has finished reviewing it. If you have an electronic copy of your portfolio, you may want to leave a copy with the interviewer at the end of the interview.

Be sure you have placed copies of all your original documents in your portfolio. Don't include sensitive or proprietary information in your portfolio, as some organizations feel free to copy your portfolio. In order to manage this, be sure you include the Statement of Originality and Confidentiality at the beginning of your portfolio.

After It's Over . . .

Take time after your interview to debrief. Were they interested in your portfolio? Did you feel rushed in presenting it? Did it stay shut in your lap during the whole interview? Think about how you used it and how you can improve. Keep these things in mind for your next interview.

Be sure to follow up with a thank-you letter to the interviewer. Thank-you letters should be relatively brief, thanking the interviewer for his or her time. Try to include some personal comment that will help the interviewer remember you. Comments about your portfolio may help jog his or her memory. If you didn't get a chance to use your portfolio in the interview and you think it could be helpful for the interviewer to see it, you might consider sending a copy of your portfolio with the thank-you letter. If you have an electronic portfolio, you might send a CD of your portfolio, or direct them to your online portfolio.

Joe's "Rejection" Letter...

Can't see the point of a thank-you letter for a rejection? Joe had an interview for a public health position on Tuesday. He had been specifically asked to apply for the position and thought the interview had gone well. He was angry and upset when he received a rejection letter in the mail on Wednesday. Nevertheless, he sent a thank-you letter, indicating that it was good to meet the interviewer and he hoped she would keep him in mind for positions in the future. The next day he received a frantic phone call from the interviewer. She told him his résumé had gotten into the wrong pile! He never should have received the letter, and he was most definitely being considered.

Thank-you's create good will and extend your presence to the interviewer. You never know when this may come back to you.

Getting the Internship Experience

Your dietetic internship experience is a particularly important part of your education. You gain practical experience while working in the dietetics field and make connections with a potential full-time employer. Your portfolio can be a valuable asset in proving your worth. It can set you apart from the other applicants and show your preparation and commitment to the field. As in a regular job interview, the organization is trying to decide why they should select you and how you can help them. As of April 15, 2004, there are 265 dietetic internships currently accredited by the Commission on Accreditation for Dietetics Education. To see details on the programs, go to: http://www.eatright.org/Public/7782_13285.cfm

The Dietetic Internship Application

When you are ready to complete your internship application, refer to your portfolio for all the details. Your portfolio contains your accomplishments, awards, activities, classes, and volunteer activities all in one place. You should have no trouble completing the application form.

You can purchase a diskette containing the application form from the ADA web site— www.eatright.org. Do a search on the site for "Supervised Practice Program Application Disk." It is well worth the nominal fee to be able to fill out the form on the computer and then print as many copies as you need.

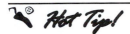

Complete your internship application on your computer. Buy the diskette containing the internship application form from the ADA web site.

Internship Interviews

Your career portfolio is also a great tool to use during internship interviews. You can use the portfolio to explain your experiences and show your work. Use it to answer questions and explain how you would be a good fit for the organization. If you are having a telephone interview, be sure to have your portfolio in front of you as you answer questions. It can give you more confidence when you can refer to your work samples, coursework, and volunteer efforts during the interview. Your portfolio can help you remember all your accomplishments and serve as a reminder of what areas you want to focus on during the interview.

Tracking Personal Goals in the Internship

You can use your portfolio to track goals and objectives you plan to achieve as an intern. You indicate the skills you want to acquire and the work that needs to be accomplished. You will use the skill assessment documents from each rotation to track your progress and document your abilities. Your internship director or preceptor will sign off on your abilities and evaluate your performance on the job.

The internship experience is an excellent way to collect work samples and certificates for your portfolio. Use your portfolio to track project timelines and chart your progress toward your goals. Contract with the internship director, telling them about your portfolio and your need for concrete work samples. You will probably find them very happy to accommodate your needs. Having an intern who is dialed into accomplishing specific goals and objectives will certainly be a positive experience for them as well!

Once You Have the Job

If you have been offered a permanent position with the employer, congratulations! You are now ready to shift your portfolio from a job-hunting tool to a professional review and promotion tool. You can use the portfolio to track your achievement on the job and progress on your professional goals.

Use the portfolio to track your quarterly and annual goals at work. Keep track of the projects you are involved in, committees you've served on, professional development seminars you have attended, and any other professional opportunities. You'll still want to track your community service involvement and any personal certifications and education you pursue on your own time.

Using the Portfolio for Reviews and Promotions

When it's time for your quarterly review, you'll want to overview your accomplishments over the last period and get your portfolio ready to go. If you've kept copies of your projects and activities during the quarter, you should be ready for your review. Tell your boss about your portfolio and offer to let him or her review it several days prior to the review. This can help the interviewer prepare better questions and have time to reflect on all your accomplishments. Sometimes it's amazing to see how much you have really accomplished! As you grow profession- ally, your goals and work philosophy will also change. Make sure you keep this updated and current.

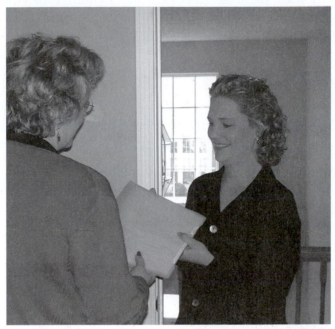

Give your portfolio to your supervisor before your review.

Now that you know how to use the portfolio during your perfor- mance review, let's talk about how to use it during the reviews where you are up for a promotion. A promotion may be a new title, new assignment to a different branch of the organization, or simply progression within the company hierarchy. In any of these cases, your portfolio should reflect your work from the period of your last promotion. If that was two years ago, then your work should reflect the last two years. If you have not been promoted yet, have your portfolio reflect your work from the time you began your employment.

Work samples, should be just that—samples—not everything you ever did. Just as in the career portfolio, you need to choose highlights of your best work. Even if something is not able to fit on an 8.5" x 11" sheet of paper, you should still include it. You might want to include a summary sheet in your portfolio and indicate that the full project is available for review. Your choices should summarize as many skills as possible and as much professional growth as possible. In these cases, it may be appropriate to include prior good reviews as evidence of your wonderful performance, which is, of course, deserving of the reward of a pay increase and/or the "corner office."

The Portfolio in Action

As you work with your portfolio in more interview settings, you'll come to appreciate how much your portfolio can add to the mix. You really can show off your skills and abilities to the best of your advantage. Once you have the job, you can transition your portfolio to track your professional life at work. Remember, your portfolio is a tool for life—your life and your career. Success!

 Taking Action!

In a job interview:

- Practice using your portfolio in an interview setting with a friend.
- Get used to your portfolio and where your samples and documents are located.
- Update your portfolio for each interview. Target your work samples to the needs of the employer.
- Use your portfolio to answer questions in the interview.

In a job review:

- Explain your portfolio and its purpose to your boss before your review.

- Check that your portfolio and work samples help to demonstrate what you have done during the past review period. Update your samples as needed.

- Give your boss your portfolio to look at ahead of the review.

- Use the portfolio in the review to demonstrate your abilities or to answer questions.

To help complete an internship application:

- Use the portfolio to help you complete the application form.

- Use your portfolio when writing the letter of application.

- Become familiar with the contents of your portfolio.

- Practice using your portfolio during an interview.

- Use your portfolio during a phone interview or physical interview.

CHAPTER 8

A MATTER OF STYLE

You are a professional, you have the credentials and the confidence to get ahead. You need to make sure your portfolio projects the same impression. If your portfolio looks sloppy and disorganized, don't even bother to take it to the interview or meeting. Your portfolio must look as clean, organized, and professional as you do.

The focus of this section is on style: the look, feel, and presentation of the materials in the portfolio. This section provides some basic guidelines for producing your work samples and other documents in your portfolio by taking a look at:

- Working with words and pictures (text and graphics)
- Production tips for video and photography
- Physical production of materials using copiers, scanners, and printers.

Text

Have you ever been reading something and suddenly you realize that you have no idea what you just read for the last four pages? This happens to all of us, but why? Are we not concentrating hard enough, or is the material boring? Your goal in creating your career portfolio is to keep the person reading it awake and interested. You need to make sure the information is easy to understand, well organized, and presented in an interesting style. You want the reader to grasp the meaning of your work without needing to read every word.

Some people write the way they talk—you can almost hear their voices. Your writing needs to have a "voice" when people read it; otherwise everything becomes just words on paper. Be yourself. Your goal is to say what you need to in your professional voice, in a clear, clean, and concise way.

Just as important as the words you use is the look and feel of the text. The following section will give you ideas for improving the style of your words.

- **Organize first—** Decide what you want to say before you begin writing.

- **Create an outline—** Outline the main ideas of what you want to say; then go into detail on each idea.

- **Use "mind mapping"—** Mind mapping is the process of writing ideas on paper, grouping words and ideas, and clustering ideas in a nonlinear format.

- **Compose at the computer—** Today, many people compose and write at the computer, since they can keyboard information faster than they can write it down on paper.

- **Have a friend take notes—** Talk to someone else and have them jot down notes. This is a great way to start getting organized.

- **Use a conversational tone—** Use a relaxed and informal style of writing. Write in first person, using I, as in I have done this ... I participated in ... I am managing ....

- **Use active vocabulary versus passive—** Active vocabulary projects the idea that you are currently working on something. Compare the use of passive words such as **does, get, show,** to active words like **doing, getting, showing**.

- **Avoid slang and too much jargon—** While it may look impressive, colloquialisms may turn what you are saying into code. Remember, the goal is to make everything clear and easy to understand.

- **Tell the truth—** It's always easier to write what you believe and what you have done versus making things up and trying to be impressive.

- **Proof your work—** Proofing your work ensures a professional look and feel to the documents you produce. Spelling, punctuation, or grammar errors can be embarrassing.

- **Use bullet points—** Bullets are an easy way to organize information in a readable, concise way. You've probably noticed after reading through this book that we, the authors, love to use bullet points. Here's a bulleted list of some of the reasons to use bullet points:

- Bullets are used to:
  - ♦ Highlight key points in the text
  - ♦ Make it easier to quickly scan through information
  - ♦ List several points or examples
  - ♦ Eliminate unnecessary text from sentences.

Now, take a look at the same information, written in paragraph form rather than using bullets and decide which is easier to read:

> Bullets pull out key information and make it easier for a reader to quickly scan through a lot of information. Bullets are often used when you are listing several points or examples. They also can eliminate unnecessary text from sentences.

Fonts

The look and style of the letters in your documents come from the fonts. Fonts are one of the simplest ways to control the look of your document and can be used to let your creativity and personality flow onto the page.

Serif vs. sans serif fonts— There are thousands of fonts available these days. All of these fonts fall into two major categories: serif or sans serif. Each of these groups has a different look and can be used to emphasize specific pieces of information in the document.

Serif fonts have the little flourishes at the ends of letters. The font you are reading now is a serif font called Bookman. Notice the curve of an "a" or the edges on a "T."

Examples of serif fonts are:

Times New Roman   Garamond   Bookman Old Style

Sans serif fonts don't have the flourishes and curves in the letters.

Examples of sans serif fonts are:

Arial   Humanist   Dom Casual   Tahoma

Decorative fonts— Be careful when you use decorative and funky fonts. These can be serif or sans serif. They are great for projects and section pages in your portfolio, but don't use them as main text in a document. They are hard to read. Use them as accent only, and never on a résumé. Examples of decorative fonts include:

Marydale   Party   Burweed ICG   Treefrog

Guidelines for Font Usage

There are no strict rules for the use of fonts, but here are some general guidelines:

- **Use serif fonts for body text**— Serif fonts are easier to read because our eyes use the little flourishes on letters to distinguish the letters. Most of the books you read are in a serif typestyle.

- **Use sans serif fonts for headings**— Sans serif fonts are often used for headings and titles rather than text. They are used to capture interest and draw attention to a particular section.

- **Use all caps sparingly— USING ALL CAPITALS CAN BE DISTRACTING AND HARD TO READ. THE USE OF ALL CAPS ON THE WEB OR IN AN E-MAIL IS THE EQUIVALENT OF SHOUTING.**

- **Don't be afraid to experiment with different fonts**— Find one that says something about your personality, be it *elegant*, **bold,** stylish, or slightly wild. Just remember, it must be readable. You don't want your reader struggling to see what the text says. If text is hard to read, we usually stop reading and skip to something else, which could cause someone to bypass some very important information about you. Consider using this type of font in the title or heading section.

- **Don't** mix too *many* fonts together *in* a document— Try to stick to one font for text and another for headings. Your work can look jumbled if you use too many variations.

- **Bold and *italic*—** The same goes for **bold** and *italic*: use them sparingly, when you need something emphasized.

- **Avoid underlining text!—** <u>Underlining is a tool that was used in the era of the typewriter, when we didn't have bold and italic.</u> Don't use it.

- **Use a proportional font—** Speaking of typewriters, have you ever noticed how every letter on a typewritten document takes up the same amount of space? Proportional fonts will take up less space, let you fit more on a page, and are easier to read. In the sample below, both paragraphs are set in 12 point size, but the nonproportional looks bigger:

```
This text is an example of a nonpropor-
tional font. Every character or space takes
up the same amount of space, and it takes a
lot of space to say something.(Courier)
```

This text is an example of a proportional font. Each character takes up as much room as it needs. (Bookman)

- **Leave only one space after a period—** Remember the typing rule about leaving two spaces after a period? Two spaces were used so you could easily see the end of a sentence in the typewriter age. With the advent of word processors and proportional fonts, we don't need the extra space. You may think it's a hard habit to break, but it is actually very easy to do.

- **Choose the correct font sizes—** The size of the font also affects the readability of the document. The most common size is 12-point. This book is written in 12-point font to make it easy to read at a glance. Ten point is the smallest size we recommend using on résumés and other documents. Any smaller, and it is very hard to read. The text in footers and headers can be smaller than 10-point, as long as they are still readable.

- **Watch the size of headings—** Most headings are printed in 16 to 18 point. Make sure your heading isn't too big for the text; meaning, don't combine 18-point headings with 10-point text.

- **Use spell check—** All good word processors contain a program to check spelling. Use this to correct typing and spelling mistakes. OK, this is an obvious step, but it's amazing how many documents we see where this simple, convenient step was overlooked. Typos look bad (especially on the front page of your portfolio!).

- **Don't rely on the spell checker—** Proof your work. Too many people rely on the spell checker to catch all their mistakes. Unfortunately the spell checker can't recognize words that are spelled correctly but misused in a sentence.

(You no that I'm talking about, don't ewe?— You **know w**hat I'm talking about, don't **you**?)

Margins, Tabs, and Spacing

The margins, tabs, and spacing you use in a document will change depending on what you are producing. Keep in mind how the document will be used when setting up the page.

Here are some general rules:

- **Single space your text—** You're probably familiar with single and double spacing. Double spacing is commonly used for reports, but single spacing should be used for most of the documents in your portfolio. Generally, you leave a double space between headings and the body of the text.

- **Use a generous margin around the page—** Allow a generous margin around your page, generally 3/4" to 1" around the entire page. Don't make your margins any smaller than 1/2", or your page will look crowded. Many people like to make notes in the margins of a résumé during an interview, and good use of white space in the form of margins allows this. Wider margins also give documents a clean and open look.

- **Don't be afraid to go to a second page—** Two or three balanced, open pages look much better than one cramped page. Keep in mind the information in your documents should be important. Don't go to two pages when you can trim out unnecessary details.

- **Get to know your word processor—** Look for the easy ways to center and indent information.

- **Keep the style consistent—** Decide on a look and style for your portfolio documents and then stick with it. Use the same margins, fonts, and spacing on these documents.

- **Use customized line spacing—** If you "get into" designing the look of your documents, you may discover that a double space after a heading is too much space. If you really want to customize your document, play with settings for the space above or below the text. This command is often found in the same location as the single- or double-spacing commands and can be used to add extra spacing before or after a heading.

Which of the following combinations looks best to you?

Work Philosophy: *(single spaced)*
I believe that every person should receive excellent customer service.

Work Philosophy: *(double spaced)*

I believe that every person should receive excellent customer service.

Work Philosophy: *(6 points)*
I believe that every person should receive excellent customer service.

Headers and Footers

Headers and **footers** are areas of text that appear at the top and bottom of a page, outside the normal space used to enter information. Headers and footers are used to print text that should appear on each page of a document, such as page numbers, dates, titles, or names. In this book, the page numbers and the chapter number and title appear in the footer. If you are planning to duplex a document (print on both sides of a page), you should use the **mirror margin** settings to have information in your headers and/or footers appear on the opposite sides of a left- and right-facing page.

Header and footer information is entered separately from regular text, and usually has tab settings preset to print information left-justified, centered, or right-justified on the page.

Text placed in a header or footer should be in a smaller font, usually 7 to 9 point. You may want to print a line between the header or footer and the main body of text to keep them separated. Here's an example of a page with footers:

Heading

a;sdlkfjaslfasd;lfkasjd;a;
a;akdjflakd;falksdlsklds
a;lskfjakjadlksjdaiejle;liej
a;lsdifasifaslfeifalea;sfehi
a;ldkfafeias;fiefnefiefnlis
a;lfiealisejlaieja fie efeifflie
;lkjlkjlsdfjaieja;lifjaelieff;
aife iefeif ejfiaef;alsife iefj
;alkjlakaieaslifefisefie asie
a;lkfjaslf slfkjsfljs ssl sf; slf
;lkjaliefj idfjle;slfekajsd;flkja

Michael Heroux   Feasibility Study
Pg. 10   4/26/04

- **Include your name and the page number on each page—**
  If your document is two or more pages, include your name
  and a page number in the header or footer of each page.

White Space

You'll hear graphic designers and desktop publishers constantly babbling about the correct use of white space. No, white
space isn't the inside of a padded cell or blizzard conditions in
the Midwest; rather, white space is the unprinted area that
appears in and around the text and graphics on a page.

When you make the margins wider in a document, you are
increasing the amount of white space on the page. Take a look
at some of the manuals and documentation you've got lying
around, and you'll see lots of variations on the use of white
space. A page which has narrow margins and lots of text can be
tiring to read. A page with too much white space can make a
reader think he or she is missing information. When possible,
add graphics and pictures to a page to add interest and give the
reader's eyes a break.

Here are some examples showing the use of white space on the page:

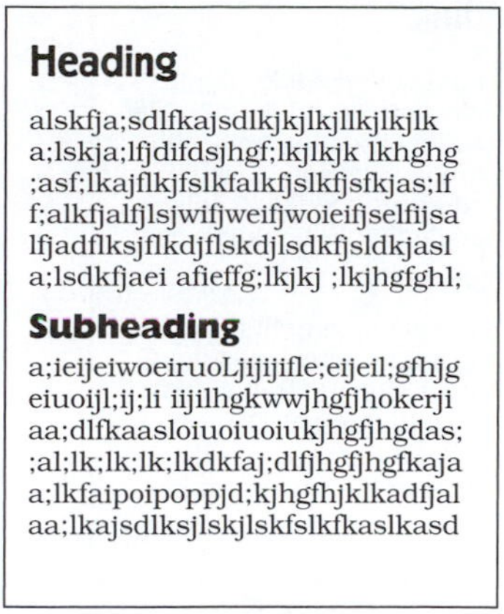

Heading

alskfja;sdlfkajsdlkjkjlkjllkjlkjlk
a;lskja;lfjdifdsjhgf;lkjlkjk lkhghg
;asf;lkajflkjfslkfalkfjslkfjsfkjas;lf
f,alkfjalfjlsjwifjweifjwoieifjselfijsa
lfjadflksjflkdjflskdjlsdkfjsldkjasl
a;lsdkfjaei afieffg;lkjkj ;lkjhgfghl;

Subheading

a;ieijeiwoeiruoLjijijifle;eijeil;gfhjg
eiuoijl;ij;li iijilhgkwwjhgfjhokerji
aa;dlfkaasloiuoiuoiukjhgfjhgdas;
;al;lk;lk;lk;lkdkfaj;dlfjhgfjhgfkaja
a;lkfaipoipoppjd;kjhgfhjklkadfjal
aa;lkajsdlksjlskjlskfslkfkaslkasd

Figure 1

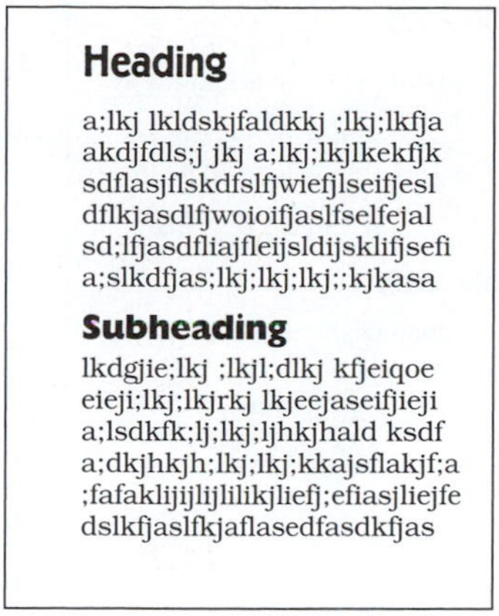

Heading

a;lkj lkldskjfaldkkj ;lkj;lkfja
akdjfdls;j jkj a;lkj;lkjlkekfjk
sdflasjflskdfslfjwiefjlseifjesl
dflkjasdlfjwoioifjaslfselfejal
sd;lfjasdfliajfleijsldijsklifjsefi
a;slkdfjas;lkj;lkj;lkj;;kjkasa

Subheading

lkdgjie;lkj ;lkjl;dlkj kfjeiqoe
eieji;lkj;lkjrkj lkjeejaseifjieji
a;lsdkfk;lj;lkj;ljhkjhald ksdf
a;dkjhkjh;lkj;lkj;kkajsflakjf;a
;fafaklijiljiliikjliefj;efiasjliejfe
dslkfjaslfkjaflasedfasdkfjas

Figure 2

Figure 1 contains very little white space and looks cramped. Compare it to Figure 2 where we added a wide left margin.

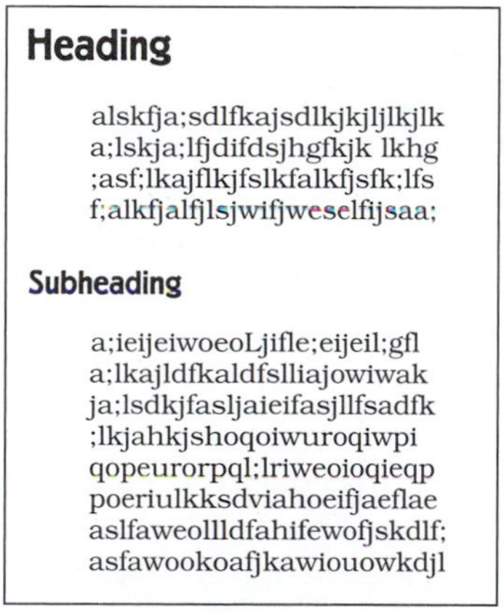

Heading

alskfja;sdlfkajsdlkjkjljlkjlk
a;lskja;lfjdifdsjhgfkjk lkhg
;asf;lkajflkjfslkfalkfjsfk;lfs
f,alkfjalfjlsjwifjweselfijsaa;

Subheading

a;ieijeiwoeoLjifle;eijeil;gfl
a;lkajldfkaldfslliajowiwak
ja;lsdkjfasljaieifasjllfsadfk
;lkjahkjshoqoiwuroqiwpi
qopeurorpql;lriweoioqieqp
poeriulkksdviahoeifjaeflae
aslfaweollldfahifewofjskdlf;
asfawookoafjkawiouowkdjl

Figure 3

Figure 3 adds side headings to the text to make the headings stand out.

Heading

alskfja;sdlfkajsdlkjkjlklkjl
jas;lskja;lfjdi;lkkjk gfas;dl
;asf;lkajflkjfsfjsfkjas;lfklfa
f;alkfjalfjljwoieifjselfijsalfi
lfjadflksjlsjlsdkfjsldkjasld
a;lsdkfjaffkj ;lkjhgfghl;aeij

Subheading

a;ieijeiwoifle;eijeil;gfhjgfge

Figure 4

Heading

a;lkj lkldsjfaldkkj ;lkj;lkf-
akdjfdls;jjkj a;lkj;lkjlkejklef
sdflasjflskfslfjwilseifjeslifja
dflkjasdlfwoioiflfijaselfejal
sd;lfjasdfk kkfjsl ljsdifjsefi
a;slkdfjaj;lkj;lkj;;kjkjk dsa

Subheading

lkdgjie;lkj ;lkjl;dlkj kjkfje
eieji;lkj;ljrkj lkjegie kjkjeji
a;lsdkfk;l;lkj;ljhkjhkjalddf
a;dkjhkjhlj;lkj;kflkajkjf;a
;fafaklijijlijilikjlief;esjliejfe
dslkfjaslfkeijasf sdsdkfjas

Figure 5

Placement of graphics is another important consideration in the use of white space. Keep pictures aligned with text or centered as in Figure 4. You can also add interest to a page by adding accent lines as in Figure 5.

Visual Media—Working with Pictures and Video

A picture is worth a thousand words. It is very important to get your pictures to look their best in order to convey the right impression. There's no question that we learn more quickly from pictures than from words on a page. Like anything else in your portfolio, pictures and videos should demonstrate your ability to perform a specific skill or competency and should be used when words won't convey this or would take too long.

Photographs

Photographs are used to emphasize your work. Take the best shots that demonstrate your work, but don't include too many photos. Photographs can be useful when you want to:

- **Display a finished product—** Displays, posters, special campaign materials, booths you have created for a health fair, etc.

- **Put your talents on display—** Public speaking, training sessions, meetings, television appearances, anywhere you are in action.

Tips for Taking Better Photographs

- **You should appear in the photo when possible—** This provides proof that it's your work, not someone else's.

- **Pay attention to film speed—** 100-speed film is good for outdoor shots where you don't need a flash. When shooting indoors, use 200- or 400-speed film and use a flash.

- **If you're working with a digital camera—** Shoot your photos at the highest quality setting. The higher the quality (resolution) of the picture, the better your print will be. You will also be able to blow up or reduce the photo and still have a good quality picture.

- **Get close—** Get close to your subject (unless you're photographing wild animals!). Use a telephoto lens to get closer if needed.

- **Fill the field—** Use the field finder on the camera and completely fill the picture with the product. Again, get close to the subject!

- **Watch where you stand—** Don't shoot pictures into light. The light meter of a camera adjusts for the brightest light, often making the real subject of the picture too dark.

- **Watch your background—** Most people look a little strange with a flower arrangement for a hat or a pole growing out of their heads!

- **Be prepared—** Try out the equipment before you have to take the picture (i.e., know how the equipment works before a critical moment, so you don't forget to take off the lens cap or find out you have dead batteries in your flash!).

- **Use a tripod—** Tripods keep your work steady and prevent blurry pictures.

- **Consider getting a special camera holder—** If you will be taking lots of still shots of products sitting on a table, make a $35 investment in a camera holder specifically designed for taking overhead pictures.

Using Video

Video can be used when you want to show examples of yourself in action. Video takes pictures and adds sound. Keep in mind that no one really enjoys watching home videos, so keep your video short, to the point, and make it worth watching. Limit your video to three-, five-, 10-, or 20-minute segments. No one is going to sit through more than a 20-minute video. Videos are usually given to an interviewer to review at a later time and are not used during the interview. Videos should be clearly labeled with your name, the content and purpose of the video, and the length.

Tips for Better Videos

- **Tips for photos also apply to video.**
- **Emphasize your skills**— Keep the emphasis of your video on your skills, not on your production abilities.
- **Be prepared**— Always test out equipment ahead of time, especially if you are borrowing the equipment. It's always good to have extra batteries and an extension cord handy.
- **Watch your lighting**— Make sure the lighting is correct.
- **Label the video**— Indicate your name, the subject, and the length of video clips.

Tips for Looking Your Best in Front of a Lens

Your looks:

- **Get a good night's rest**— Weariness and stress are visible. Makeup can only cover so much. You want to avoid shiny foreheads and noses.
- **Make sure your hair looks neat and attractive**— If you need a haircut, get one several days in advance.
- **Gentlemen, be careful shaving, avoid scrapes and cuts**— Watch out for "five o'clock shadow."
- **Women**— Wear makeup as usual. If you wear heavy liner on your lower eyelid—go lightly or avoid it so you do not look like a raccoon.

Clothing choices:

- Wear a proper fitting suit and shirt.

- Darker tones make the body look thinner.
- Avoid navy blue. It shows everything and appears murky.
- Avoid wearing black and white in color photos.
- Avoid turtleneck shirts and sweaters.
- Avoid wearing a white shirt. It can produce a glare.
- Wear a suit jacket for a serious look. Button the top button on all double-breasted suits.
- Make sure your clothes are not too tight. If you have recently gained weight, a new larger shirt will mask the gain better than a tight-fitting outfit.
- Neckties should look conservative unless the tie is part of a uniform look.
- Keep your jewelry to a minimum.

Production Tools—Copiers, Scanners, and Printers

Copiers, scanners, and printers are the most common tools you'll use to produce your portfolio. Here are some tips for making their output look as good as possible.

Copiers

- **Clean the machine**— Take a bottle of glass cleaner and a cloth with you the next time you go to make copies. Clean the glass on the machine and your final copies will be much clearer.
- **Align the paper**— Center the page on the copier and make sure the paper is straight on the copier. Nothing is more annoying than crooked copies!
- **Enlarge small fonts**— If the original document is in 10 point or smaller type, enlarge it to make it easier to read.

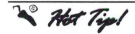

Clean copying machines, scanning beds, and any electronic equipment with flat glass screens using glass cleaner before copying to ensure quality.

- **Copying small pieces of paper—** If you're copying something smaller than 8.5" by 11", be sure to put a white piece of paper behind the document so the background is clear. If necessary, tape the original to the paper to hold it centered. If you are trimming the copy from a larger size, be sure to use scissors. Think neat.

- **Color copying—** Color copying can be expensive. Look at the project and determine where you need color in your work samples. Use color copying when you want to accent something special. Certificates, awards, PowerPoint slides, and photos are good choices for color copying.

- **Consider scanning as an alternative—** While you can use a color copier to copy photographs, the quality may not be as good as you would like. Consider scanning color pictures for higher quality and then printing them on photo paper with a high quality color printer.

- **When in doubt, ask for professional help—** The staff at copy centers are usually happy to assist you with your copying.

Scanning Equipment

- **Flatbed scanners—** Flatbed scanners are becoming a low-cost way of making color copies with your computer. Multifunction ink jet printers that can scan, copy, print, and fax are popular choices for home printers.

- **Scanning is often a good alternative to photocopying—** It can produce a clearer picture. Combined with a color printer, it can also be a cheap alternative to color copying.

- **Resolution—** Scanning is measured in dpi—dots per inch. The higher the dpi, the more detailed and sharper the picture or document. Use no less than 300 dpi, preferably 600 dpi or higher, when scanning.

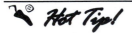

When scanning documents, set your resolution to 300 dpi minimum. They may take up more disk space, but the quality of your printout will be much better!

- **Scan certificates and degrees**— For a better look, consider scanning certificates and degrees; they copy official seals better than a copier.

Paper and Printing

Paper

As you choose the paper you'll use in your portfolio, keep in mind that the main purpose of the paper is to enhance the text and graphics in the document, making it easier to read. It can also be used to distinguish you from other people and can capture a bit of your style. Here are some guidelines for selecting paper:

- **Use high-quality, 24-lb. paper**— Heavier weight paper has a better feel and look. It also helps keep printing from showing through to the other side.

- **Don't use fax paper or any type of thermal paper**— Thermal paper will fade and age. Make copies of any faxes.

- **Paper color**— Use subtle colors, nothing harsh. Use the same paper consistently throughout the portfolio. Use color to draw attention to items you want to emphasize or to title pages. Don't overuse colored paper; limit yourself to a maximum of three different colors. White should be your primary color. Make sure your résumé is printed on white paper.

Printing

- **Use a high-quality printer**— Good printers can produce 300- to 600-dpi (dots per inch) resolution. The higher the dpi, the higher the quality of the document.

- **Working with inkjet printers**— If you are printing on an inkjet printer, use paper that's been designed for inkjets, or paper that says it's compatible. Inkjet paper is designed to absorb the ink and give you a clearer, sharper image than regular laser jet paper.

Tabs and Cards

Here are some ideas to keep in mind when creating the tabs and work sample overview cards used in the portfolio:

- **Buy standard size products—** Avery brand labels are the most popular brand. Most word processors can automatically set up a document based on common sizes of Avery brand labels. If you buy another brand of labels, be sure they have the same label measurements as the Avery brand. Most word processing packages have preset templates which lay out the page's margins and space. Setting up labels can be as simple as entering a number from the box. Check out the supply list in chapter 9, "Resource Guide," for specific product numbers.

- **Watch the product's box to see if it is designed for laser or inkjet printers—** If you are printing on an inkjet printer, get the product designed for the inkjet. It is usually brighter and has a coating designed to hold the ink and dry very fast. The ink may spread on products designed for the laser printer. In general, laser and inkjet products are interchangeable, but don't go to all that work only to find out that the end product looks sloppy.

Follow the guidelines in this chapter and you're sure to have a fantastic looking portfolio! Putting the effort into making your portfolio look professional will pay off in your interviews and reflect the quality back onto you.

Send Us Your Success Story

Our research continues. We are interested in your stories about using a portfolio. We want to hear your experiences and opinions. Tell us how your friends and family reacted. Let us know what you did to improve the portfolio's layout or contents. Share with us how you used the portfolio with your employer and how your organization reacted.

We are interested in the types of work samples you used and how you produced quality copies. Tell us what you would like to see developed or improved in the portfolio. Our next book will have expanded coverage of the electronic portfolio. If you have any questions, ideas, or comments we would love to hear them. Let us know how we can help.

Please send your success story to:

Learnovation® LLC
My Portfolio
PO Box 502150
Indianapolis, IN 46250

or e-mail us at: **portfolio@learnovation.com**

Visit our web page to learn more about career mechanics and other people's portfolio experiences.

http://learnovation.com

 Taking Action!

Things to do:

- Proof the documents in your portfolio. Check for spelling and grammar errors.

CHAPTER 9

RESOURCE GUIDE

This resource guide contains the following materials designed to help make the development of your career portfolio easier:

1. **Supply List** - Materials to purchase.

2. **Emergency Instructions for Portfolio Assembly** - When you need to put together a portfolio fast.

3. **Action Verbs** - A list of verbs used when describing what you have done. Typically used on your résumé and in goal setting.

4. **Department of Labor SCANS** - A listing of general skills and competencies. Useful when setting up skill sets and looking up résumé language.

5. **Transferable Skill List** - A listing of skills you can use in many different jobs and situations.

6. **Common Job Titles and Skills in Dietetics** - A chart of common job titles and the skills needed for each position. Use this chart when you are looking for keywords, planning goals, and searching for work samples.

7. **Dietetic Work Samples** - A chart of possible work samples for common skill areas in a dietitian's portfolio.

8. **Common Dietetics Professional Abbreviations** - A listing of acronyms commonly used in the dietetic profession.

9. **Sample Dietetic Internship Application** - A completed dietetic internship application.

10. **List of Templates on CD** - A listing of the files included on the CD that accompanies this book.

1. Supply List

Take this list with you to the office supply store. You can also find these items on the Internet at **www.officemax.com** or **www.officedepot.com** or **www.staples.com.** Visit **www.learnovation.com** for complete portfolio kits containing all the supplies needed to create your portfolio.

- **Plastic file tote box or accordion folder** (1)
- **Hanging file folders, standard file size** (20–30)
- **Zippered three-ring notebook** (preferably leather or simulated leather).

Sheet Protectors

- **Clear sheet protectors** (50–100) Different weights are available:

  Avery 74130 - Diamond Clear© Sheet Protectors - Super Heavy-weight, Top Loading - 50 sheets per box.

  Avery 75530 - Diamond Clear© Sheet Protectors - Standard Weight, Top Loading - 25 sheets per package.

  Avery 74097 - Diamond Clear© Sheet Protectors - Economy Weight, Top Loading - 75 sheets per package.

- **Connected sheet protectors** (3–5 sets):

  Avery 74301 - Bound Sheet Protector Sets - Clear, 10-page set.

  Avery 74300 - Bound Sheet Protector Sets - Clear, 5-page set.

- **Multi-capacity sheet protectors—** If you want to include a magazine or a project that you would pull out of the sheet protector to view, you can purchase multi-capacity sheet protectors which can hold 50 pages in each protector.

  Avery 74171 - Multi-capacity Sheet Protectors - 25 sheets per package.

  Avery 74172 - Multi-capacity Sheet Protectors - 10 sheets per package.

- **Fold out sheet protectors—** These sheet protectors hold an 11" x 17" sheet of paper or two 8.5" x 11" side by side.

  Avery 75256 - Fold Out Sheet Protectors - 5 sheets per package.

- **8.5" x 11" plastic photo sheet holders** (2–3 as needed):

  Avery 13403 - Photo Pages - Eight 3-1/2" x 5" photos per page.

  Avery 13407 - Photo Pages - Four 3-1/2" x 5" horizontal photos per page.

  Avery 13406 - Photo Pages - Four 4" x 6" horizontal photos per page.

  Avery 13401 - Photo Pages - Six 4" x 6" photos per page.

Tabs

There are several types of tabs available: Tabbed sheet protectors, extra-wide paper dividers, or self-adhesive tabs. (1-2 sets)

- **Tabbed sheet protectors:** You can insert a title page into each tabbed page

  Avery 74160 - Protect 'N Tab ™ Tabbed Sheet Protectors - Clear 5-Tab, Single Set

  Avery 74110 - Protect 'N Tab ™ Tabbed Sheet Protectors - Clear 8-Tab, Single Set

- **Extra-wide paper dividers:**

  Avery 11221 - Worksaver® Extra WideTM BIG TAB Insertable Tab Dividers - Laser/Ink Jet, 5-Tab Clear, 3-hole punched

  Avery 11222 - Worksaver® Extra WideTM BIG TAB Insertable Tab Dividers - Laser/Ink Jet, 8-Tab Multi color, 3-hole punched

  Avery 11223 - Worksaver® Extra WideTM BIG TAB Insertable Tab Dividers - Laser/Ink Jet, 8-Tab Clear, 3-hole punched

  Avery 11220 - Worksaver® Extra WideTM BIG TAB Insertable Tab Dividers - Laser/Ink Jet, 5-Tab Multi color, 3-hole punched

- **Self-adhesive tabs:**

  Avery 16282 - Printable Self Adhesive Tabs - 1 3/4" x 1".

Additional Materials

- **Blank sheets of business cards** (10 sheets)

  Avery 08371 - Ink Jet Business Cards - White, 10 cards per sheet

  Avery 08471 - Ink Jet Business Cards - White, 10 cards per sheet

  Avery 05911 - Laser Business Cards - White, 10 cards per sheet

- **Nameplate or vinyl card holder**

  Avery 73720 - Self-Adhesive Business Card Holders - for 3-1/2" x 2" business cards

- **Paper (high quality)**

  For inkjet printing: use 24# bright white paper.

2. Emergency Instructions for Portfolio Assembly

I Need a Portfolio Now!!!

"Oh, it won't take that long to put it together."

"I have one that I used last time."

"My interview is tomorrow and I have to do all this before I can start on my portfolio?"

"Do I update my portfolio, or do I sleep and shower?"

If you've just purchased this book and want to put together a portfolio for an interview tomorrow morning, or if you've had this book for a while and suddenly your interview is upon you, there's still hope. Based on several frantic experiences of our own, rest assured you can put together a basic career portfolio in three hours if you have a computer, printer, and your best friend's help.

Run to the Office Supply Store and Buy . . .

- Zippered three-ring binder
- Clear page protectors (a box or two of 50)
- Extra-wide page tabs
- Plastic stick-on business card holder for front of portfolio
- High quality paper
- Extra ink cartridge (if you're using an inkjet printer).

Grab Your Best Friend and . . .

- Your box of work samples or file of projects
- A computer and printer
- Your most recent résumé.

We can't stress enough the importance of having a friend help you with the assembly process. Friends can help you make wise choices for work samples, determine your management philosophy and goals, stuff paper into page protectors, make up tabs and exhibit cards, and help you through this somewhat frantic time. A good friend serves as a sounding board and tends to ask questions of you that you wouldn't think of yourself.

Include These Sections in Your Portfolio

- Work Philosophy
- Career Goals
- Résumé
- Skill Areas— Determine different areas. Place work samples in appropriate areas.
- Letters of Recommendation (if available)
- List of Professional Membership and Awards
- Community Service— Any work samples and letters available
- References.

Don't Forget to . . .

- Create tabs for each section
- Make up work sample overview cards for your work samples on plain paper.

See Chapters 2 to 4 for specific guidelines for each of these sections.

3. Action Verbs

Action verbs are used in your résumé to indicate the types of actions you have done. Action verbs can be used in present tense to indicate things you are currently doing.

Accomplished	Equipped	Ordered
Achieved	Established	Organized
Adapted	Evaluated	Paid
Adjusted	Expanded	Performed
Administered	Expedited	Persuaded
Advanced	Filed	Planned
Analyzed	Furthered	Presented
Assessed	Gained	Prioritized
Assisted	Generated	Processed
Authorized	Guided	Produced
Budgeted	Handled	Provided
Built	Helped	Recommended
Chaired	Implemented	Reduced
Combined	Improved	Repaired
Communicated	Increased	Reported
Completed	Initiated	Researched
Composed	Instructed	Reviewed
Conducted	Interviewed	Revised
Coordinated	Introduced	Screened
Created	Learned	Served
Delegated	Led	Set up
Designed	Located	Simplified
Developed	Maintained	Strengthened
Directed	Managed	Supervised
Displayed	Maximized	Supported
Edited	Modified	Taught
Employed	Monitored	Trained
Encouraged	Motivated	Typed
Enhanced	Negotiated	Updated
Enlarged	Operated	Wrote

4. Department of Labor SCANs

Here is a list of baseline skills and competencies established by the Department of Labor, known as SCANS. Use this skill list to review and organize your own skill sets or to assist in writing your skill descriptions for your résumé.

The Foundation—Competency Requirements:

Basic Skills
- Reading
- Writing
- Arithmetic
- Mathematics
- Speaking
- Listening.

Thinking Skills
- Thinking creatively
- Making decisions
- Solving problems
- Seeing things in the mind's eye
- Knowing how to learn
- Reasoning.

Personal Qualities
- Individual responsibility
- Self-esteem
- Sociability
- Self-management
- Integrity.

Competencies—Effective Workers can Productively Use:

Resources
- Allocating:
  - time
  - money
  - materials
  - space
  - staff.

Interpersonal Skills
- Working on teams
- Teaching others
- Serving customers
- Leading
- Negotiating
- Working well with people from culturally diverse backgrounds.

Information
- Acquiring and evaluating data
- Organizing and maintaining files
- Interpreting and communicating
- Using computers to process information.

Systems
- Understanding social, organizational, and technological systems
- Monitoring and correcting performance
- Designing or improving systems.

Technology
- Selecting equipment and tools
- Applying technology to specific tasks
- Maintaining and troubleshooting technologies.

From SCANS—Secretaries' Commission on Achieving Necessary Skills. 1991, U.S. Department of Labor

5. Transferable Skill List

Verbal Communication

- Perform and entertain before groups
- Speak well in public appearances
- Confront and express opinions without offending
- Interview people to obtain information
- Handle complaints in person over phone
- Present ideas effectively in speeches or lecture
- Persuade/influence others to a certain point of view
- Sell ideas, products, or services
- Debate ideas with others
- Participate in group discussions and teams.

Nonverbal Communication

- Listen carefully and attentively
- Convey a positive self-image
- Use body language that makes others comfortable
- Develop rapport easily with groups of people
- Establish culture to support learning
- Express feelings through body language
- Promote concepts through a variety of media
- Believe in self-worth
- Respond to nonverbal cues
- Model behavior or concepts for others.

Written Communication

- Write technical language, reports, manuals
- Write poetry, fiction, plays
- Write grant proposals
- Prepare and write logically written reports
- Write copy for sales and advertising
- Edit and proofread written material
- Prepare revisions of written material
- Utilize all forms of technology for writing
- Write case studies and treatment plans
- Demonstrate expertise in grammar and style.

Train/Consult

- Teach, advise, coach, empower
- Conduct needs assessments
- Use a variety of media for presentation
- Develop educational curriculum and materials
- Create and administer evaluation plan
- Facilitate a group
- Explain difficult ideas, complex topics
- Assess learning styles.

(continued)

Plan and Organize

- Identify and organize tasks or information
- Coordinate people, activities, and details
- Develop a plan and set objectives
- Set up and keep time schedules
- Anticipate problems and respond with solutions
- Develop realistic goals and action to attain them
- Arrange correct sequence of information and actions
- Create guidelines for implementing an action
- Create efficient systems
- Follow through, ensure completion of a task.

Counsel and Serve

- Counsel, advise, consult, guide others
- Care for and serve people; rehabilitate, heal
- Demonstrate empathy, sensitivity, and patience
- Help people make their own decisions
- Help others improve health and welfare
- Listen empathically and with objectivity
- Coach, guide, encourage individuals to achieve goals
- Mediate peace between conflicting parties
- Knowledge of self-help theories and programs
- Facilitate self-awareness in others.

Create and Innovate

- Visualize concepts and results
- Intuit strategies and solutions
- Execute color, shape, and form
- Brainstorm and make use of group synergy
- Communicate with metaphors
- Invent products through experimentation
- Express ideas through art form
- Remember faces, accurate spatial memory
- Create images through sketches, sculpture, etc.
- Utilize computer software for artistic creations.

Interpersonal Relations

- Convey a sense of humor
- Anticipate people's needs and reactions
- Express feelings appropriately
- Process human interactions, understand others
- Encourage, empower, advocate for people
- Create positive, hospitable environment
- Adjust plans for the unexpected
- Facilitate conflict management
- Communicate well with diverse groups
- Listen carefully to communication.

Leadership

- Envision the future and lead change
- Establish policy
- Set goals and determine courses of action
- Motivate/inspire others to achieve common goals
- Create innovative solutions to complex problems
- Communicate well with all levels of the organization
- Develop and mentor talent
- Negotiate terms and conditions
- Take risks, make hard decisions, be decisive
- Encourage the use of technology at all levels.

Management

- Manage personnel, projects, and time
- Foster a sense of ownership in employees
- Delegate responsibility and review performance
- Increase productivity and efficiency to achieve goals
- Develop and facilitate work teams
- Provide training for development of staff
- Adjust plans/procedures for the unexpected
- Facilitate conflict management
- Communicate well with diverse groups
- Utilize technology to facilitate management.

Financial

- Calculate, perform mathematical computations
- Work with precision with numerical data
- Keep accurate and complete financial records
- Perform accounting functions and procedures
- Compile data and apply statistical analysis
- Create computer-generated charts for presentation
- Use computer software for records and analysis
- Forecast, estimate expenses and income
- Appraise and analyze costs
- Create and justify organization's budget to others.

Administrative

- Communicate well with key people in organization
- Identify and purchase necessary resource materials
- Utilize computer software and equipment
- Organize, improve, adapt office systems
- Track progress of projects and troubleshoot
- Achieve goals within budget and time schedule
- Assign tasks and sets standards for support staff
- Hire and supervise temporary personnel as needed
- Demonstrate flexibility in crises
- Oversee communication, e-mail.

Analyze

- Study data or behavior for meaning and solutions
- Analyze quantitative, physical, and/or scientific data
- Write analysis of study and research
- Compare and evaluate information
- Systematize information and results
- Apply curiosity
- Investigate clues
- Formulate insightful and relevant questions.

Research

- Identify appropriate information sources
- Search written, oral, and technological information
- Interview primary sources
- Hypothesize and test for results
- Compile numerical and statistical data
- Classify and sort information into categories
- Gather information from a number of sources
- Patiently search for hard-to-find information
- Utilize electronic search methods.

Construct and Operate

- Assemble and install technical equipment
- Build a structure, follow proper sequence
- Understand blueprints and architectural specs
- Repair machines
- Analyze and correct plumbing or electrical problems
- Use tools and machines
- Master athletic skills
- Landscape and farm
- Drive and operate vehicles
- Use scientific or medical equipment.

from Life Work Transitions.com

©1999–2002 by Deborah L. Knox and Sandra S. Butzel, Butterworth-Heinemann

6. Common Job Titles and Skills in Dietetics

Adapted from: U.S. Department of Labor Bureau of Labor Statistics, "*Occupational Outlook Handbook, 2004 - 2005 Edition*" Available from www.bls.gov.

Dietary Manager

Alternate Job Titles:	corporate account manager; director of nutrition; school food service director

Key Skills and Performance Areas
- Directs and coordinates food service activities
- Food service operations manager
- Ensures menus and department policies conform to nutritional standards, government/establishment regulations and procedures
- Quality control of patient diet management
- Plans and coordinates standards and procedures of:
  - Food storage
  - Preparation
  - Service
  - Equipment and department sanitation
  - Employee safety
  - Personnel policies and procedures
- Deploys food safety, sanitation, and quality standards
- Interacts with institutional administration to improve food service
- Computes operating costs
- Dietetic competency certificate.

Food Service Dietitian

Alternate Job Titles: food service manager

Key Skills and Performance Areas

- Overall operation of establishment including:
  - Purchase food
  - Select and plan menus
  - Oversee staffing of kitchen and dining room operations
  - Maintain health, safety and sanitation levels.
- Establish standards for personnel performance, service to customers, menu rates, and advertising and publicity
- Purchase food and equipment
- Inspect the premises to maintain health, safety and sanitation regulations
- Estimate cost of food and beverage
- Requisition or purchase supplies
- Interact with customers and vendors
- Perform detailed clerical and financial duties such as:
  - Directing payroll operations
  - Handling large sums of money
  - Taking inventory
- Supervise a sales and advertising staff in large establishments
- Handle problems and cope with the unexpected and daily tasks.

Chief Clinical Dietitian

Alternate Job Titles: clinical nutrition manager; dietitian; administrative director in dietetics department

Key Skills and Performance Areas

- Administers, plans, and directs activities of a health-care center's nutrition department
- Establishes policies and procedures, and provides administrative direction for:
  - ◆ Menu formulation
  - ◆ Food preparation
  - ◆ Food service
  - ◆ Purchasing
  - ◆ Food safety and sanitation
  - ◆ Staffing and scheduling
- Hires dietetic staff, RDs, DTRs, and other necessary staff
- Directs departmental education programs
- Coordinates interdepartmental professional activities
- Consults management on matters pertaining to dietetics.

Clinical Dietitian

Alternate Job Titles: registered dietitian; long-term care dietitian; outpatient dietitian; pediatric dietitian, medical nutrition therapist

Key Skills and Performance Areas

- Plans therapeutic diets
- Implements preparation and service of meals for patients
- Consults with physician and other health-care personnel to determine nutritional needs and diet restrictions
- Formulates menus for therapeutic diets based on medical and physical conditions of patients
- Integrates patients' menus with basic institutional menus

- Inspects meals served for conformance to prescribed diets and for standards of palatability and appearance
- Instructs patients and their families in:
  - Nutritional principles
  - Dietary plans
  - Food selection
  - Food preparation
- May engage in research
- May teach nutrition and diet therapy to medical students/hospital personnel
- May hold special certifications.

Consultant Dietitian

Alternate Job Titles: **institutional nutrition consultant**

Key Skills and Performance Areas
- Advises and assists personnel in public and private establishments in food service systems and nutritional care of clients
- Makes recommendations for conformance level that will provide nutritionally adequate, quality food
- Plans, organizes, and conducts orientation and in-service educational programs for food service personnel
- Develops menu plans
- Assesses, develops, implements, and evaluates nutritional-care plans and provides for follow-up
- Ability to write proposals and reports
- Consults with health-care team concerning nutritional care of client
- Confers with designers, builders, and equipment personnel in planning for building or remodeling food service units
- Negotiates personal salaries and contracts
- Writes business plans and proposals
- Utilizes business and entrepreneurial skills.

Research Dietitian

Alternate Job Titles: research nutritionist; clinical research dietitian

Key Skills and Performance Areas

- Conducts nutritional research to expand knowledge in one or more phases of dietetics
- Plans, organizes, and conducts programs in nutrition, foods, and food service systems, evaluating and utilizing appropriate methodology
- Studies and analyzes recent scientific discoveries in nutrition for:
    - Application in current research
    - Development of tools for future research
    - Interpretation to public
- Communicates findings through reports and publications.

Teaching Dietitian

Alternate Job Titles: dietetic internship director; cooperative extension educator; public health nutritionist; didactic program director; preceptor; professor (assistant, associate, or full)

Key Skills and Performance Areas

- Plans, organizes, and conducts educational programs in dietetics, nutrition, and institution management for dietetic interns and nutrition majors; may include nursing students, and other medical personnel
- Develops curricula
- Prepares manuals, visual aids, course outlines, and other material used in teaching
- Instructs students on:
    - Principles of nutrition
    - Menu planning
    - Medical nutrition therapy

- ◆ Food service operations
- ◆ Food cost control
- ◆ Marketing
- ◆ Administration of dietary department
- ■ May engage in research.

Dietetic Technician

Alternate Job Titles: **None**

Key Skills and Performance Areas

- ■ Provides services in assigned areas of food service management
- ■ Teaches principles of food and nutrition
- ■ Provides dietary consultation under direction of dietitian
- ■ Plans menus based on established guidelines
- ■ Standardizes recipes and tests new products for use in facility
- ■ Supervises food production and service
- ■ Obtains and evaluates dietary histories of individuals to plan nutritional programs
- ■ Guides individuals and families in food selection, preparation, and menu planning, based upon nutritional needs
- ■ Assists in referrals for continuity of patient care
- ■ May select, schedule, and conduct orientation and in-service education programs
- ■ May develop job specifications, job descriptions, and work schedules
- ■ May assist in implementing established cost control procedures.

7. Dietetics Work Samples

Work samples are more than continuing education attendance. This is a list of possible work samples for common work sample categories.

Tabbed Area of Portfolio	Possible Work Samples
Patient Education	■ Patient handouts ■ Preservation materials ■ Web research ■ Patient comprehension forms ■ Feedback sheets.
Food Service	■ Menu(s) you have designed ■ Food safety certification ■ Patient satisfaction ■ Photos of yourself working in the kitchen ■ Standard operating procedures developed ■ List of equipment you can operate with your supervisor's sign off.
Management	■ Schedules written ■ Performance evaluations ■ Forms you have created to assist staff ■ Committee reports and presentations.
Finance	■ Purchasing forms ■ Portion control systems developed ■ Inventory systems created ■ Budgets developed ■ Forecasts developed.
Clinical	■ Nutrient calculation sheets ■ Software applications you are trained on ■ Patient assessment forms ■ Patient consultation forms.
Research Methods	■ Methodology ■ Reports written ■ Photos of poster presentations ■ Publications ■ Proposals written.

8. Common Dietetics Professional Abbreviations

(Compiled by Kyle Shadix)

ADAF	ADA Foundation
BOD	Board of Directors
BSN	Bachelor of Science in Nursing
CADE	Commission on Accreditation for Dietetics Education
CCC	Certified Chef de Cuisine
CCE	Certified Culinary Educator
CEC	Certified Executive Chef
CD	Certified Dietitian
CCN	Certified Clinical Nutritionist
CDE	Certified Diabetes Educator
CDM	Certified Dietary Manager
CDHCF	Consultant Dietitians in Health Care Facilities DPG
CDN	Certified Dietitian Nutritionist
CDR	Commission on Dietetic Registration
CNM	Clinical Nutrition Manager
CNSD	Certified Nutrition Support Dietitian
COE	Council on Education
COP	Council on Practice
CP	Coordinated Programs
CPI	Council on Professional Issues
CSP	Certified Specialist in Pediatric Nutrition
CSR	Certified Specialist in Renal Nutrition
DBC	Dietitians in Business and Communications DPG
DCE	Diabetes Care and Education DPG
DDPD	Dietetics in Development and Psychiatric Disorders DPG
DEP	Dietetic Educators of Practitioners DPG
DHHS	Department of Health and Human Services
DMA	Dietary Managers Association

(continued)

DNS	Dietitians in Nutrition Support DPG
DPG	Dietetic Practice Group
DT	Dietetic Technician
DTR	Dietetic Technician, Registered
EdD	Doctor of Education
FADA	Fellow of The American Dietetic Association
FCP	Food and Culinary Professionals DPG
FNCE	Food and Nutrition Conference and Exhibition
GN	Gerontological Nutritionists DPG
HEN	Hunger and Environmental Nutrition DPG
HOD	House of Delegates
JCAHO	Joint Commission on Accreditation of Healthcare Organizations
JADA	Journal of The American Dietetic Association
LD	Licensed Dietitian
LDN	Licensed Dietitian/Nutritionist
LN	Licensed Nutritionist
LNC	Legislative Network Coordinator
LPPC	Legislative and Public Policy Committee
LTC	Long-Term Care
MBA	Master of Business Administration
MEd	Master of Education
MMSc	Master of Medical Science
MNS	Master of Nutritional Science
MNT	Medical Nutrition Therapy
MPA	Master of Public Administration
MPH	Master of Public Health
MTS	Master of Theology Studies
NCND	National Center for Nutrition and Dietetics
NE	Nutrition Entrepreneurs DPG
NNM	National Nutrition Month

NST	Nutrition Support Therapist
ON	Oncology Nutrition DPG
PhD	Doctor of Philosophy
PN	Pediatric Nutrition DPG
QA	Quality Assurance
QM	Quality Management
RYDY	Recognized Young Dietitian of the Year
SCAN	Sports, Cardiovascular, and Wellness Nutritionists DPG
RD	Registered Dietitian
SPRC	State Professional Recruitment Coordinator

9. Sample Dietetic Internship Application

The following section contains portions of a dietetic internship application. Look at the different sections that are required and how you can use the information in your career portfolio when filling out the application.

SUPERVISED PRACTICE PROGRAM APPLICATION

All information on this application must be typed.

Date: January 30, 2002

Name	Budgazad	Sari	
	(Last)	(First)	(Middle or Maiden)

Present Address

	(Street)	(Apt #)	
	(City)	(State) (Zip Code)	(Phone)

Permanent Address

	(Street)		(Apt #)
	(City)	(State) (Zip Code)	(Phone)

Telephone number where you can be reached on day of appointment

Area Code

Social Security Number

Foreign Applicants: Designate Immigration Status _____ **Expiration Date:** _____

Supervised Practice Entrance Date Preferred August 12, 2002

Full-Time Full-Time **or Part-Time (if applicable)** _____

Actual or Expected Date Baccalaureate Degree Will Be/Was Conferred May 2002

Actual or Expected Date Didactic Program in Dietetics (DPD) Requirements Will Be Completed May 2002

Education: List all colleges and universities attended, with most recent listed first.

School	Address (City/State)	Dates	Degree
University of Delaware	Newark, DE	Fall 1998- Spring 2002	Bachelor of Science
Syracuse University	Syracuse, NY	Sep 1997-Jun 1998	
Adelphi University	Garden City, NY	Sep 1997-Jun 1998	
New York Institute of Technology	Old Westbury, NY	Jan 1997-May 1997	

Prepared by The American Dietetic Association and Dietetic Educators of Practitioners Practice Group for optional use by dietetics education programs. (1998)

Basic contact and school information comes from your résumé.

Recommendations: List the names of all individuals who will complete your recommendation forms.

Name	Title	Address	Phone
Dr. Connie Vickery	Professor, Nutrition & Dietetics		
Dr. Marie Kuczmarski	Professor, Nutrition & Dietetics		
Beth Webb	Registered Dietitian		
Dr. Cheng-Shun Fang	Professor, Nutrition & Dietetics		

Extracurricular/Volunteer Activities: List memberships (specify year(s) of membership), appointed or elected offices you held in organizations. Volunteer activities not related to dietetics.

September 2001	Coordinated benefit concert and raffle for WTC Red Cross Disaster Relief Fund		University of Delaware
Fall 2000-present	President	Nutrition & Dietetics Club	University of Delaware
Fall 2000-present	Member	Eating Disorder Coordinating Council	University of Delaware
Fall 1999-present	Public Relations Chair	Delaware Undergraduate Student Congress	University of Delaware
Spring 1999-present	Member	American Dietetic Association	
Spring 2000	Reporter for school newspaper, *the Review*		University of Delaware
Spring 2000	Assistant Broadcaster, Student Life Television		University of Delaware

Honors: List scholarships and honors received.

Winter 2002- Research Study in Hawaii: *Honors Section* NTDT 475 Transcultural Food Habits

Fall 2001- Selected speaker by Department of Nutrition & Dietetics to represent Class of 2002 at Spring Convocation

December 2000- Received university recognition for undergraduate research on end-stage renal disease and nutrition supplementation

March 2000- Honored nutrition student at university's annual Women of Promise Dinner

February 2000- Kappa Omicron Nu National Honor Society for Nutrition & Dietetics Students who exhibit excellence in research, scholarship, and leadership; **1998-2001** Deans List; **1998** National Society of Collegiate Scholars Award

Graduate Record Exam Score: Date
(if applicable) Taken _____ Verbal _____ Quantitative _____ Analytical _____

Undergraduate Coursework:
Cumulative grade point average based on 4.0 system __3.8__

Grade Point Average for DPD course work based on 4.0 system __3.72__

*Recommendations are from your list of references.
Extracurricular/volunteer activities are your professional
memberships and non-dietetic volunteer experiences.
Honors are your scholarships and awards received.*

Paid work experience in the past 5 years (you may include work experience in the past 10 years if applicable to your situation): List paid work experience beginning with the most recent experience. Do not list experiences that were part of required practicum/field experience. Briefly describe responsibilities.

Organization Name City/State	Position, Title	Inclusive Dates (Mo/Yr)	Hrs/Wk	Name and Title of Supervisor/Phone #
1. University of Delaware Newark, DE	Community Educator	Sep '00- Dec '01	3 Hrs/Wk	Juan Villamarin, Chairperson Anthropology

Key Responsibilities
- Conducted a lecture session on healthy eating strategies to students enrolled in anthropology course
- Designed a nutrition project for male and female college students using three-day food records
- Assisted in research to compare college students' dietary behaviors with national food surveys
- Completed nutrient analyses of students' recorded diets using *Food Processor* software

2. MBNA America Bank Wilmington, DE	Nutrition & Corporate Health Promotion Intern	Jun-Aug '01	40 Hrs/Wk	Beth Webb, R.D.

Key Responsibilities
- Composed internet articles for MBNA health newsletter
- Designed educational displays for health resource libraries and coordinated monthly health fairs
- Tracked program participation data in the following areas: nutrition & weight control, cholesterol, blood pressure, diabetes, osteoporosis, smoking cessation and maternal and infant health
- Conducted individual nutrition counseling under supervision of R.D. & performed health risk appraisals on MBNA population

3. Temple Beth El Hebrew School Newark, DE	Foreign Language teacher	Feb '00-May'01	10 Hrs/Wk	Ann Herman, Director

Key Responsibilities
- Taught concepts and grammar of Hebrew language to middle school students
- Introduced literature, research projects, ethnic foods, music, & culture
- Participated in planning of assemblies and student performances

4. University of Delaware Student Health Services Newark, DE	Assistant to Registered Dietitian	Feb-May '99	3 Hrs/Wk	Sandy Baker, R.D./

Key Responsibilities
- Responsible for internet research and application of diet analysis software
- Prepared appropriate pamphlets and calorie counters for patients
- Developed menus and nutrition fact sheets for distribution to college students

5. Kid Mazeum Cedarhurst, NY	Hostess	Sep 1996- Sep 1998	20 Hrs/ Wk	Ivy Robinson

Key Responsibilities
- Coordinated and responsible for preparation of events including food, music, and décor
- Handled reception involving retail and contract agreements

Use additional pages as needed.

The paid work experience section from your résumé.
Use the keywords from your résumé to list the key responsibilities.

Volunteer experience related to dietetics in the past 5 years: List volunteer experience related to dietetics, beginning with most recent experience.

Organization Name City/State	Position, Title	Inclusive Dates (Mo/Yr)	Hrs/Wk	Name and Title of Supervisor/Phone #
1. University of Delaware Newark, DE	Nutrition Peer Mentor	Feb '02- present	6 Hrs/ Wk	Charlene Hamilton, Associate Professor Nutrititon & Dietetics

Key Responsibilities — Interpret current, scientific-based nutrition information for consumers (students)

Use the Internet to research current topics in nutrition

Become familiar with resources available to students who request information about

dietary supplements, diet & weight loss management, and other nutritional concerns

Distinguish between scientifically sound and fraudulent nutrition information

2. University of Delaware Nutrition & Dietetics Club Newark, DE	President (member)	Sep '00- present Sep '98- present	5 Hrs/ Wk	Dr. Marie Fanelli Kuczmarski, Professor Nutrition & Dietetics

Key Responsibilities — Coordinate annual health fair celebrating National Nutrition Month

Arrange and direct cooking demonstrations at dormitories

Compose and distribute newsletters that promote healthy living

3. Skyline Middle School Wilmington, DE	Food & Nutrition Science Alliance, Coordinator	Oct '01- present (2x / Mth)	6 Hrs/ Wk	Maggie Gimmel, Director

Key Responsibilities — Present food models to educate middle school students on using the Food Guide Pyramid

Participate in customized nutrition education sessions to promote "5-A-Day For Better Health"

Conduct question & answer period with students concerning nutrition related topics

4. Head Start Elkton, Maryland	Volunteer	Nov '00-present (2x / Mth)	2 Hrs/Wk	Mrs. Lynn Wellmaker, Director

Key Responsibilities — Direct cooking demonstrations and coordinate nutrition-related activities at local Head Start

Teach about healthy snacks and seasonal foods

5. Alfred I. Dupont Children's Hospital Wilmington, DE	Volunteer	Nov '00-present (1x / Mth)	3 Hrs/Wk	Laura Mitchell, Child Life Specialist

Key Responsibilities — Participated in visits to pediatric oncology unit of hospital

Used arts and craft to teach about foods related to national holidays (i.e. Thanksgiving)

Use additional pages as needed.

Volunteer experience is very important when applying for a dietetic internship. Use your résumé and volunteer work samples to complete this section.

Volunteer experience related to dietetics in the past 5 years: List volunteer experience related to dietetics, beginning with most recent experience.

Organization Name City/State	Position, Title	Inclusive Dates (Mo/Yr)	Hrs/Wk	Name and Title of Supervisor/Phone #
6. University of Delaware Newark, DE	Guest Speaker for Department of Nutrition & Dietetics	Nov '01 Apr '01, Oct '00	1 Hr / event	Dr. Connie Vickery
Key Responsibilities	Guest Speaker at undergraduate Nutrition Seminar: promoted events conducted by the Nutrition & Dietetics Club & shared personal nutrition-related work experiences Guest Speaker at Women's Health Conference: conducted a lecture session on a variety of topics including: healthy eating habits, the benefits of folic acid, and weight loss strategies Guest Speaker at New Student Orientation: oriented freshmen and transfer students enrolled in the Nutrition & Dietetics Program			
7. University of Delaware Newark, DE	Project designer, Eating Disorder Coordinating Council	Sep-Dec '00 Member: Sep '00-present	2 Hrs/ Wk Meetings: 1 Hr/ Wk	Nancy Nutt, Program Coordinator Center for Council & Student Development
	Designed "Love Your Body" door hangers to promote positive body image on campus Used computer graphics to create messages concerning behavioral & psychological health Participate in event planning for fundraisers and wellness fairs			
8. Delaware Food Bank Newark, DE	Volunteer	Nov '99 (2x/ Mth)	3 Hrs/ Wk	Lisa Carlisle
Key Responsibilities	Toured the facility and learned about the "community kitchen" Organized canned foods and donated products for distribution to local facilities			
9. New York University Medical Center New York, NY	Volunteer	June '99	5 Hrs/ Wk	Eydie Cole, M.S., R.D.
Key Responsibilities	Shadowed a Registered Dietitian during daily hospital rounds Assisted in nutrition counseling for cardiac patients and attended nutrition education sessions			
10. Brandeis School Cedarhurst, NY	Kitchen Aide	May- June '99	10 Hrs/Wk	Michelle, Director of Cafeteria Services
Key Responsibilities	Learned to handle school food service operations including: food procurement, preparation, and menu planning Prepared and served lunch foods to early childhood and elementary school students			

You can find volunteer experiences from your involvement in organized events, demonstrations, presentations, written articles, non-paid experiences, and school events.

Sample Dietetic Internship Application (cont.)

Professional Courses: (Include all courses in foods, nutrition, community nutrition, nutrition education, nutrition counseling, nutrition and disease, foodservice systems, management, computer courses, etc.). Use additional pages as needed. Identify with a (X) if courses included a lab or practicum component.

Courses to Meet DPD Requirements

College or University	Course Title	Lab/ Practicum	Course No.	Term &Year	No. of Credits	Grade Earned	Grade Points Earned
University of Delaware	HNRS: Nutrition Concepts		NTDT 200	98 F	3	A-	11.000
University of Delaware	Introduction to Nutrition Professions		NTDT 103	99 S	1	Pass	0
University of Delaware	Food Principles		NTDT 201	99 F	2	A	8.000
University of Delaware	Food Principles Lab	X	NTDT 211	99 F	1	A	4.000
University of Delaware	Introduction to Clinical Dietetics		NTDT 240	00 S	3	A-	11.000
University of Delaware	Food Science		FOSC 305	00 S	3	A	12.000
University of Delaware	Quantity Food Prod and Service		NTDT 321	00 F	3	A-	11.000
University of Delaware	Lab: Quantity Food Production & Service	X	NTDT 325	00 F	1	A	4.000
University of Delaware	Food Service Facility Design		NTDT 328	00 F	1	A	4.000
University of Delaware	Macronutrients		NTDT 400	00 F	3	A	12.000
University of Delaware	Management of Food & Nutrition Services		NTDT 322	01 S	3	A	12.000
University of Delaware	Micronutrients		NTDT 401	01 S	3	A	12.000
University of Delaware	Nutrition and Disease		NTDT 440	01 S	3	A	12.000
University of Delaware	Dietetics Seminar		NTDT 403	01 F	1	Pass	0
University of Delaware	Nutritional Assessment Methods	X	NTDT 421	01 F	3	A	12.000
University of Delaware	Community Nutrition		NTDT 460	01 F	3	A-	11.000

Additional Courses completed:

College or University	Course Title	Lab/ Practicum	Course No.	Term &Year	No. of Credits	Grade Earned	Grade Points Earned
University of Delaware	HNRS: Nutrition Controversies		NTDT 222	99 S	1	A	4.000
University of Delaware	Independent Study Undergrad. Teach Asst.		NTDT 366	00 S	1	A	4.000
University of Delaware	Independent Study End-Stage Renal Disease		NTDT 366	00 F	2	A	8.000
University of Delaware	Indep. Study Nutrition/ Health Promotion Internship		NTDT 466	01 F	3	A	12.000

Totals: Credits 42   Grade Points Earned 164

Grade point average in above courses (divide grade points earned by no. of credits): 3.90

Refer to your Academic Plan of Study and your transcript for the courses and grades you have taken.

Sari Budgazad
Letter of Application

February 7, 2002

New-York Presbyterian Hospital
New York Weill Cornell Medical Center
525 East 68th Street
New York, NY 10021

Dear Dietetic Internship Evaluation Committee,

My interest to pursue a dietetic internship through New York Presbyterian Hospital reflects the knowledge and experiences I acquired over the past four years. Advancing through a didactic program has motivated me to seek unique opportunities in research, leadership, and communications. I feel that my academic skills have provided me with the incentive to create nutritional awareness and promote healthy lifestyle changes among various populations. After devoting time to distributing food at community centers, conducting nutrition education lessons at elementary schools, and directing health fairs at local organizations, I learned that work itself becomes a reward.

Assuming roles outside the academic setting have exposed me to a myriad of experiences related to the dietetics profession. My interpersonal skills have expanded through my involvement in developing health promotion programs and speaking at nutrition seminars. As a health promotion intern at MBNA America bank, I aided in directing the Creating Health Awareness Motivates People (C.H.A.M.P.) program for employees with physical and mental disabilities. From distributing apples at the company cafeteria to accompanying employees on fifteen-minute walks, I incorporated the benefits of healthy food choices and aerobic activity in a fun, creative, and comprehensive manner. In addition, I assisted in corporate skin cancer screenings, and menu planning customized for patients on low-fat, low-sodium diets. Through health and prevention expositions, I grew committed to implementing programs that encouraged employees to develop their personal dimensions of wellness. I shared my experiences in a presentation to an undergraduate seminar as a way of inspiring other students to pursue education through professional opportunities in nutrition.

Many organizations require a letter describing why you are interested in applying for the internship position. This organization required the letter to be handwritten. This statement will be easier to complete after you have gone through the process of creating your own career portfolio.

Page 2

As president of the University of Delaware Nutrition and Dietetics Club, I learned to handle multiple tasks and grow as an effective leader. While taking initiative to plan events that promoted nutrition across the lifespan, I recognized the need to delegate responsibilities in order to bring projects to closure. Coordinating health fairs during National Nutrition Month and participating in the Food and Nutrition Science Alliance illustrate activities achieved through teamwork. During the health fair last March, I used creativity to stimulate interest in nutrition-related topics. As a way of increasing calcium intake among college students, nutrient information was presented in the form of healthy snack samples (i.e. yogurt and calcium-fortified cereal) and "Got Milk?" posters. Moreover, I used food models to educate adolescents on estimating serving sizes without a measuring cup and following a balanced diet. Both events featured nutrition displays designed to communicate dietary messages that coincided with the needs of the target population.

I feel that my personal background has provided me with insight and awareness of my responsibility to the field of medical nutrition therapy. My food choices are strongly influenced by a blend of Mediterranean and Western European culture, which have encouraged me to explore transcultural food habits. While studying abroad in Hawaii, I interacted with indigenous populations and observed their dietary practices. The significance of adapting to a variety of people and situations is manifest in my ability to understand and educate individuals with specialized dietary needs. While working at a corporate health office, I interviewed a patient diagnosed with high blood cholesterol. In order to devise an effective meal plan, I utilized her cultural dietary practices as a means of setting goal-directed behaviors. As a result, I incorporated Indian recipes and vegetarian foods to improve the nutritional quality of her diet. By recommending spices and seasonings in substitution for flavorings high in saturated fat,

Letter of application (continued)

Use your work philosophy and goals in the letter. You can also look through your work samples to pull out and mention some of your best accomplishments in your dietetic career.

I motivated her to lose weight as well as lower her LDL cholesterol.

The value of research in the dietetics field has encouraged me to pursue independent study. I learned to utilize systematic research methods while conducting a comprehensive literature review on the topic of end-stage renal disease. The experience challenged me to explore the impact of nutritional supplementation and prepare a written report for health care practitioners. As a researcher, I have also taken initiative in designing nutrition projects within the University of Delaware anthropology department. The use of food records as a dietary assessment tool enabled me to analyze eating patterns among male and female college students. Consequently, I learned that awareness of our own food systems reflects what we eat and where our foods come from.

The relevance of using nutrition assessment methods in both clinical care and community environments is apparent through my volunteer work. During one experience, I shadowed a dietitian at NYU Medical Center. Observing her modify diets for cardiac patients reinforced my desire to learn diet assessment techniques. In the academic environment, I have studied the role of nutrition in disease management, analyzed patient case studies, and devised nutrition care plans. However, it was not until I became exposed to planning and implementing patient meals in a hospital setting that I began to truly appreciate the applied aspect of medical nutrition therapy. Furthermore, volunteering at the University of Delaware Employee Wellness Center provided me with valuable work experience in a community setting. Under the supervision of a community nutritionist, I assumed an active role in launching weight management programs, conducting health risk appraisals on Cholesterol Screening day, and designing a nutrition showcase on the topic of "Food Portion Distortion." A unique aspect of this field experience involved my interaction with a variety of staff members who demonstrated their expertise

Letter of application (continued)

Don't forget to include information on your work experiences, memberships, and volunteer efforts.

Page 4

in fitness, nutrition, and marketing. My contributions demonstrated my ability to use effective communication skills to increase employee participation rates in physical activity programs such as "30 Minutes in Motion," as well as nutrition counseling sessions. As a result, I learned to value teamwork and accept constructive criticism.

A dietetic internship that offers individualization of experience based upon my personal goals will direct me towards achieving professional objectives as a Registered Dietitian. The visual media I use to educate others has inspired me to accept new challenges that emphasize variety, proportionality, and moderation, principles that fall within the framework of the Food Guide Pyramid. As a dietetic intern, I intend to spend proportionate amounts of time exploring diverse areas in clinical, community, and research settings. In addition, I anticipate working with healthy individuals in moderation with people who require special diets because of diseases or conditions that interfere with normal nutrient requirements. Concurrent with supervised clinical practice, I feel that experience at the New York Presbyterian Womens Health Clinic will train me with skills needed to assess nutrition resources and perform nutrition evaluations in an ambulatory care setting. Eventually, I plan to specialize in community nutrition and assume a media role in the area of preventive health. Delivering quality nutrition services, networking with health care professionals, and reacting continually to misinformation to combat nutrition quackery illustrate the public relations aspect of my career goals.

I am confident that the New-York Presbyterian Hospital Dietetic Internship will motivate me to interface with diverse populations in a multidisciplinary setting. As a future dietetics practitioner, communicating credible nutrition information to help the public make informed health decisions is an intriguing pursuit!

Sincerely,

Avu Buddurzad

Letter of application (continued)

10. List of Templates on the CD

The accompanying CD contains files to help you save time while creating your career portfolio. Use these documents as a starting point. Customize these files and make them work for you. Feel free to change the fonts and rearrange information as needed. Each file was created in Microsoft Word 2000.

Faculty_Employer bios.doc - A contact list of people who are mentioned in your portfolio.

Memberships.doc - A listing of your professional memberships.

Recommendation request.doc - A sample letter for requesting a recommendation letter.

References.doc - List your references and their contact information.

Skillset.doc - A blank skill set serves as a starting point for creating checklists of your skills.

Stmt of originality.doc - A basic statement indicating that the portfolio is your property and should be respected.

SWOT Analysis.doc - A worksheet designed to help you plan your career.

Work philosophy and goals.doc - List your work philosophy and career goals.

Work sample overview cards.doc - Business card layout for printing overview cards used to identify work samples and materials in your portfolio.

Directory: e_portfolio - HTML pages that can be edited to create your own electronic portfolio. Files include:

default.htm (home page)	skill_area3.htm
philosophy_goals.htm	skill_area4.htm
resume.hm	community_service.htm
skill_area1.htm	awards.htm
skill_area2.htm	

INDEX

ADDITONAL PORTFOLIO RESOURCES

NOW AVAILABLE!

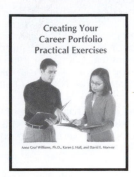

Creating Your
Career Portfolio
Practical Exercises

Anna Graf Williams, Ph.D., Karen J. Hall, and David E. Morrow

Creating Your Career Portfolio: Practical Exercises Workbook

(© 2003 Learnovation®, LLC) 128 pages. A new companion guide to the Career Portfolio series. This workbook provides nine exercises to guide you through the process of creating your career portfolio. In this book you will take a look at your skills and life experiences and begin to track your experiences, collect and organize your work samples, and discover new skills you didn't know you had. $21.95

Exercises included
1 – Your Career Portfolio Planner
2 – Auditing Job Advertisements for Skills
3 – Class Skills Inventory
4 – Transferable Skills Inventory
5 – Soft Skills Inventory
6a – Planning for the Skills You Need – College Plan of Study
6b – Planning for the Skills You Need – Jobs
6c – Planning for the Skills You Need – Transferable Skills
7a – Résumé Development – Résumé Organizer
7b – Résumé Development – Using Keywords in Your Résumé
8 – Gathering, Sorting, and Refining Work Samples
9 – Creating Your Career Portfolio – Assembly Checklist

Audio Tape

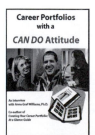

Career Portfolios
with a
CAN DO Attitude

An interview
with Anna Graf Williams, Ph.D.

Co-author of
Creating Your Career Portfolio:
At a Glance Guide

Career Smarts—Career Portfolios with a CAN DO Attitude!

This audio tape features an interview with Anna Graf Williams, overviewing the contents of a Career Portfolio and the process of creating and assembling a portfolio. Anna focuses on how to select your best work samples, use your transferrable skills to your advantage, and get that job, raise, or promotion you deserve.
45 min. $15.95

Portfolio Kits

Looking for a fast and easy way to create a portfolio? If browsing through an office supply store isn't your favorite thing, you're in luck! We have three different kits containing all the items needed to create a career portfolio with impact! - We offer three versions of the career portfolio kit: Basic, Standard, and Deluxe.

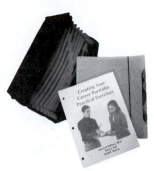

Each kit comes with a copy of Creating Your Career Portfolio: Practical Exercises.

Basic Portfolio Kit - $28.95
- Plastic 3-ring binder box w/clip
- 10 sheet protectors
- One sheet of blank business card (10 cards total)

Standard Portfolio Kit - $34.95
- Tabbed, zippered accordion file for quick organization
  of materials
- Self-closing 3-ring notebook with five tabs
- 25 sheet protectors
- Three blank business card sheets (10 cards each)

Deluxe Portfolio Kit $64.95
- Zippered 3-ring cloth binder
- 50 sheet protectors
- One plastic business card holder for cover ID
- Two 3" x 5" photo holder sheets
- One connected sheet protector set
- Two 5-set tabbed sheet protectors
- Two high capacity sheet protectors
- Three blank business card sheets (10 cards each)

FACULTY- CALL FOR SPECIAL PRICING ON PORTFOLIO KITS!

Visit our website at **www.learnovation.com**
Call 1-317-577-1190 or **fax your order to 1-317-598-0816**
Toll-Free 1-888-577-1190

CAREER PORTFOLIO VIDEOS

Career Portfolios are changing the way people interview by helping people plan, organize, and document their work samples and skills. Using a portfolio can help you get a job, get a higher starting salary, show transferable skills, track personal development, and position you for advancement.

Now, three videos are available to help you make the most of your portfolio. Each tape features advice and tips from the experts and takes a look at how real people use portfolios to advance their careers.

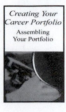

Creating Your Career Portfolio – Assembling Your Portfolio

This video overviews the career portfolio process and focuses on gathering supplies, work samples, and materials to include in a career portfolio. This video features interviews with professionals and students who have used the portfolio, tips from the experts, and detailed guidelines for putting together your own portfolio. 25 min. - $99.

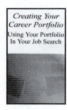

Creating Your Career Portfolio – Using Your Portfolio in Your Job Search

Once you have created your personalized career portfolio, how do you actually use it in an interview? This video features sample interviews and expert commentary to show the do's and don'ts of portfolio use in an interview setting. Learn tips on using the portfolio to your best advantage. 25 min. - $99.

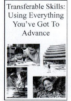

Transferable Skills – Using Everything You've Got to Advance

Learn how to identify and use your transferable skills to advance your career. This video focuses on how you can use the same skills in different areas of your life. 25 min. - $129

Buy Videos #1 and #2 for $179 and get a free copy of the At-a-Glance Guide! Three-video set with a free At-a-Glance Guide book. - $299

TO ORDER

Visit our website at **www.learnovation.com**
Call 1-317-577-1190 or **fax your order to 1-317-598-0816**
Toll-Free 1-888-577-1190

Mail orders to:
Learnovation® LLC
PO Box 502150
Indianapolis, IN 46250

Shipping:
$0-$99 - 7%
$100 and over - 6%
Indiana State Residents, please
   add 6% sales tax